Barstool Body

invisible home gym

the original

BACKPACK GYM

by

Shawn Arnold

Visit us on the web at **www.barstoolbody.com**

ISBN-13: 978-1468188981
ISBN-10: 1468188984

To my three awesome children
Chance, Caden, and Connor.
You are the inspiration which drives me
to make healthy lifestyle choices.

Table of Contents

Notice and Disclaimer

The purpose of this book is to provide you with information to help you develop exercise and dietary programs that will fit into your schedule and individual fitness level. Therefore the information provided should be viewed as supplemental information to proper exercise and dietary programs. Neither the exercise information nor the dietary information provided in this book is intended to replace or substitute any exercise or diet prescribed by your doctor. The exercises and dietary recommendations provided in this book should not be attempted without first consulting your doctor.

The editors, publishers, and authors of this book advise you the reader to follow proper safety guidelines before attempting any of the exercises in this book. Additionally, the do-it-yourself exercise equipment instructions throughout this book do not recommend any particular manufacturer or brand of equipment and therefore we advise you to take necessary precautions to ensure the safety of your own equipment. You should not attempt any exercise nor should you use any equipment that is unsafe.

The editors, publishers, and authors of this book will not be held responsible for injuries and/or damages caused by your attempt to perform the exercises, dietary recommendations, or other information provided in this book. It is your responsibility to ensure your own personal safety as well as the safety of your surroundings and people around you. You should be sure that all of your equipment is well maintained, free from defects, and safe for use.

As with any exercise program there is inherent risk of injury when performing the exercises in this book. Whether that risk is due to the specific movement required by the exercise or due to the equipment used to perform the exercise it is your responsibility to

"Give me a B"

First to all of the spelling bee champions and English grammar teachers who are reading I want to apologize for my misspelling throughout of the noun *bar stool*. To be honest, I'm not sure if the noun is supposed to be handled as a single term or as a noun phrase with the *bar* portion of the phrase acting as an adjective for the noun *stool*.

Additionally, I've utilized the privilege of combining the two separate nouns, bar and stool, by removing the space in between them to create the proper noun *Barstool* with a capital "B".

Although that may be appropriate and it probably won't cost me any points with the grammar teachers, I've also abused the privilege in other areas where the proper use of the term should be referenced as the two-separate-word term. But in light of the book's title and the name of my company, as the author I've invoked the right of author's prerogative and have chosen to refer to a bar stool throughout this book as simply barstool with a lowercase "b".

Chapter 1

"Look Dad, no hands!"

Find your motivation

When the nurse finished taking my blood pressure the perplexed look on her face spoke volumes and her, "Let's try taking that again." response didn't do much to ease my suspicions. Apparently, even though I didn't feel any different and I was only in my early thirties my body was responding to my unhealthy lifestyle choices and alerted the nurse and my respective doctor to the fact that something wasn't right. I had been diagnosed with prehypertension which was a huge smack in the face that if I didn't do something about it I was at a huge risk for high blood pressure.

My doctor was very encouraging and didn't try to push medication as the only answer. He did mention that sometimes medication is inevitable and is necessary no matter how well you take care of yourself, but he took the time to talk with me about other options. We talked about my exercise habits which at the time were fairly sparse. He also told me a story about some time he had spent with monks whom he explained had the ability to control their blood pressure through extreme self control. Now as awesome as that sounded I knew I would never have the time to perfect or even attempt that technique. Additionally, I didn't want to devote the amount of time exercising that traditional mentality concerning weight-loss suggested was necessary.

Working full-time and raising 3 kids left very little time in the day for me to spend on me and my attempts to fit conventional exercise into my regular routine just didn't work. I even began bicycling to work and joining the local bicycle club for weekly rides. But again with 3 kids and their activities it was difficult to bicycle regularly for an extended period of time.

What could I do to stretch at least another hour out of my day?

As it turns out, I really didn't need to add more time to my day, I simply needed to make a few adjustments to the way I was spending the 24 hours that I'd been given. Besides, even if had tapped into Einstein's brain waves and figured out a way to bend time and space in such a way that I could squeeze in an extra hour or two if I didn't have some sort of a plan I would have easily filled those extra hours with more stuff that provided absolutely no benefit to a healthier happier me.

Find Your Motivation

Taking the first step and starting something new is not something that comes easily to most of us. We become comfortable and complacent and lack the motivation to truly want to change. Other times we might even be discouraged enough to think that things are just going to always be the way they are and there's no sense even trying to make a change. It isn't until we are truly motivated to make a change that we step out into the unknown and open ourselves up to new possibilities.

Think back to when you were a kid learning to ride a bike. It wasn't an easy task. And despite the countless scrapes and bruises you didn't give up. Why? You were motivated to learn to ride that bike. Now fast forward a few years to when you first learned to drive. Again the task was not an easy one and if you sat down and thought about it, it was really quite dangerous. Especially the first time you ventured out onto the freeway.

I remember first learning to drive on the interstate. It was extremely frightening and I wasn't sure I could do it. So why did I? Motivation.

Although the motivating factors might have been a little different for each of us, the possibilities which were opened as a result of learning to ride a bike and learning to drive on the interstate made it easier to deal with the temporary pain of the scrapes and bruises and fears of sharing the roads with 30 ton big rigs traveling at supersonic speeds.

For me the motivation to change my lifestyle habits came when I received the news that I was at risk for high blood pressure.

If you look at my "Before" picture to the right, it's obvious that I wasn't in shape. Well, I suppose I was in some sort of shape, but it definitely wasn't good. However, what you can't tell from that picture is that I had been fairly active prior to and even during the time that picture was taken. I mean this was taken during the time I had been bicycling to work and joining my local bike club at least once a week for longer rides. Well, to be fair I've never been a huge fan of cold weather cycling and so I had taken a bit of a sabbatical during the winter months when that picture was taken. But regardless of the particular circumstances, I thought I was in pretty good shape.

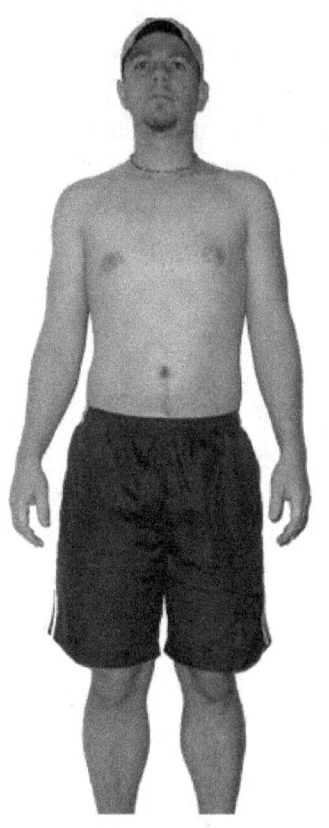

Before

I considered myself to be an active adult primarily because of my bicycling affinity. But apart from that my three kids kept me busy with all sorts of activities, not to mention the amount of effort it takes to simply keep up with and care for them in their daily routines. I would go outside and shoot some hoops. I'd rally up the neighborhood kids for a game of touch football or street baseball. I setup a net at the park across the street and held badminton tournaments. I'd march through the woods behind our house mimicking some sort of military battle. I'd go for bicycle rides through the neighborhood hauling my daughter in her bicycle seat. The activities seemed endless, but they weren't enough to fend off the monster in the closet.

As you can see I didn't have a lot of free time to devote to exercise unless I wanted to wake up at 4am. And that definitely wasn't going to happen as I value every second of sleep I can get! So going to the gym wasn't really an option. And to make matters worse, I love to eat. Junk food, high calorie breakfasts, and hamburgers were staples in my diet and quite frankly I wasn't willing to give them up. So this whole change of lifestyle to get healthy really wasn't looking like it was going to be much fun, or for that matter, something that I was willing to endure. Therefore, I decided to do a little research and formulate a plan that would fit into my lifestyle.

So what was I to do?

Part of my problem was due to the lack of physical activity during the winter months, but that lack of activity combined with less than ideal dietary habits during the holiday season was a recipe for disaster!

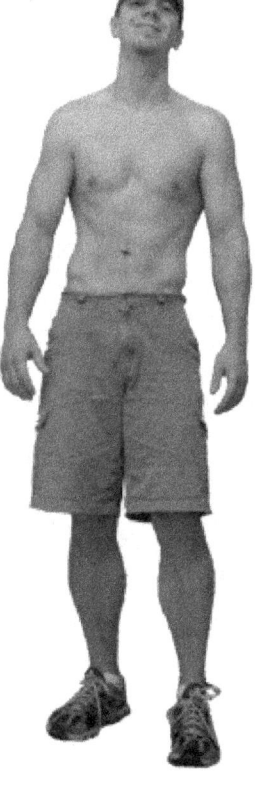

I began to evaluate my daily routine, lifestyle choices, and eating habits and along the way I noticed something that seems to contradict common sentiment concerning exercise.

After

As I began to pay more attention to the things I was doing, I was also beginning to notice the lifestyle choices and habits of the people around me. For instance I was surrounded by relatively active people such as myself. I had an acquaintance who didn't seem to notice that he was in his 50's and could probably run circles around 95% of the population. He was constantly out in his yard working. He would run a thousand miles a day and every weekend he would pack up his mountain bike or kayak and venture off to the mountains or the river. Yet despite his extremely active lifestyle choices and overall physical fitness when he went shirtless...let's just say he was storing up a few more calories around his midsection than were entirely necessary for him to make it through the winter.

And he wasn't the only one!

Several of the guys who rode in the weekly group rides were amazing cyclists who could ride 40 miles without breaking a sweat. However, if you were to pass them in the cookie aisle at the grocery store you would most likely think to yourself, "Dude keep walking unless you want to look like that guy!"

So what was my big, "Aha?"

Well quite simply it was the realization that being active wasn't going to be enough for me to reach my ultimate goal of a healthier trimmed down me. To elaborate a little, I discovered that going through the motions day after day of the same activities was going to do very little if anything at all towards helping me achieve my goals. In fact it almost seemed pointless.

Chapter 2

"Do you know your number?"

Achieve noticeable results with minimal effort in
the shortest amount of time possible.

Have you ever wondered if you are getting the maximum benefits from your workouts or if you are just wasting your time and efforts? Since the major principle of this book is to develop an exercise program that provides noticeable results with minimal effort in the shortest amount of time possible, I've given much thought to it and I'm guessing the thought has crossed your mind at some point as well. Even if the thought has never occurred to you, I feel that I would be doing you a huge injustice if I didn't tell you about one of the most valuable tools you should have in your backpack.

Before I discuss the tool, please bare with me as I lay out a few basic ground rules. Especially if you've tried using this tool previously, but couldn't quite figure out how to use it effectively.

1. As I mentioned at the onset of this book, it is of utmost importance that you evaluate your current physical condition and check with your doctor before starting any of the exercise programs or attempting to perform any of the moves or procedures described in this book.

2. Determine your unique number. This value will be based on several factors unique to your current physical condition. This might best be determined by your doctor, so when you are being evaluated in step 1 above ask your doctor to help you determine your number.

3. As your fitness level improves, reevaluate your number and adjust it accordingly.

4. Make it as simple as simple as possible, otherwise you won't use it effectively.

5. Use it to achieve results, fast!

OK, so what is this super tool? Well, the tool isn't necessarily a tangible item with material and physical properties, but rather it is a measurement and subsequent technique(s) to perform the measurement. And the value you are concerned with measuring is your heart rate (HR).

"Keep it Simple"

While obtaining your heart rate may not require any special equipment or at least anything more complex than a simple time keeping device such as the second hand on a watch you will most likely find that a heart rate monitor will make the task much easier. And if you haven't noticed it by now a reoccurring theme throughout this book has been to keep things as simple as possible. In fact it is my opinion that the most important principle one should embrace when starting something new is the old acronym KISS, "Keep It Simple Shawn" or something like that. Conveniently my first name begins with the letter S so I'm able to substitute it into last position of the acronym.

If you choose to purchase a heart rate monitor, and I would highly recommend it, there are several options available ranging in price from under ten bucks all the way up to several hundred dollars. I realize that one of the goals of this book is to provide you with a means to build an exercise system that not only fits into your lifestyle, but one that also fits into your budget and preferably as one that is inexpensive or even free. It is precisely for that reason that I mention a heart rate monitor is not required for you to measure your performance effectively. However, I want to stress once again that it will make the measuring process a lot less cumbersome.

That being said, I would not recommend going out and spending several hundred dollars on a heart monitor. In fact you should be able to find a feature rich unit in the thirty to fifty dollar range. And if you catch a break on eBay you might even score one for much less.

I mentioned previously that there are some heart rate monitors available for less than ten bucks, but these usually require you to hold your finger on a sensor built into the watch to measure your heart rate. Again, this will probably work just fine, but it will be a little more laborious than a unit which continuously displays your heart rate on your wrist which can be checked at a glance.

Therefore I would recommend that you look for a heart rate monitor in the lower-middle range, cost-wise. These will usually be comprised of two-piece units: a wrist-watch like receiver/display and a sensor/transmitter the straps around your chest.

If you find that you enjoy working out at night or if it is more convenient for you to fit your workouts into the evening or night hours it is highly likely that you will spend some time outside after dark. In this case it is import to be able to read the display of your heart rate monitor. As I alluded to in guideline 4 above, if you can't easily read the display of your heart rate monitor, you will either not use it or you will not use it effectively. Therefore you might want to purchase a heart rate monitor with a back lit display or one with a button you can press to light the display. Another option and possibly a more practical one because it will also help with overall visibility and will help to make you more visible to people around you would be to purchase a LED headlamp. These come in various sizes and styles and in multiple LED configurations. They even make them specifically for runners, however, those seem to be smaller and underpowered compared to some of the larger LED headlamps with multiple LED bulbs.

"I've got a heart rate monitor, now what?"

Now that you have your fancy new gizmo, what are you going to do with it? Well, the first thing you need to do is determine your target heart rates. There are several methods available for determining these rates and I've created a table in the Appendix to help you find your target heart rate.

Determine your resting heart rate. The best way to obtain an accurate resting heart rate it to measure your heart rate when you first wake up in the morning. Measure it as soon as you can after waking, before you situp and exert yourself in any manner. Do this for several mornings and then calculate the average for all of the mornings included in your test period.

For example if your resting heart rates for days 1, 2 and 3 are 77 beats per minute (bpm), 71 bpm, and 74 bpm respectively your average resting heart rate will be:

$(77 + 71 + 75) / 3 = 74$ bpm

A typical resting heart rate will be between 60 and 90 beats per minute.

Calculate your maximum heart rate. Probably the most accurate way to obtain your maximum heart rate is to go through a cardiac stress test under the supervision of your doctor. However, a widely accepted method to determine your maximum heart rate is to subtract your age from 220 referred to as your age-predicted maximum heart rate. For example if you are 40 years old your age-predicted maximum heart rate is:

$220 - 40 = 180$ bpm

Obviously, this doesn't take into account your particular fitness level or genetics which when factored into the equation might adjust this number by a factor of 10 or more in either direction. But for most the simple age subtraction calculation is probably close enough. However, this should not be viewed as a substitute for an evaluation by your physician.

Calculate your heart rate reserve. This is simply the difference between your maximum heart rate and your resting heart rate.

Heart Rate Reserve = Maximum Heart Rate – Resting Heart Rate

Continuing our example:

Heart Rate Reserve = 180 – 74 = 106 bpm

Calculate your target heart rates. Target Heart Rates are sometimes referred to as Training Heart Rates and refer to a range of heart rates that correspond to various levels of aerobic exercise. These are sometimes broken up into zones such as one might find on the dial of a treadmill. For these rates you have several options. One of the most common and effective options is the Karvonen Method.

Karvonen Method

This method seeks to find your target heart rate range by calculations based on 50 to 85% intensity.

Target Heart Rate 1 = ((Heart Rate Reserve) x 0.50) + Resting Heart Rate
Target Heart Rate 2 = ((Heart Rate Reserve) x 0.85) + Resting Heart Rate

To make it a little more clear lets plug in the sample heart rates we've been working with. For example:

Target Heart Rate 1 = ((180 – 74) x 0.50) + 74 = 127 bpm
Target Heart Rate 2 = ((180 – 74) x 0.85) + 74 = 164 bpm

So based on this method you will receive the maximum benefits from your aerobic exercise by keeping your heart rate between Target Heart Rates 1 and 2 or for the purpose of our example, between 127 and 164 bpm.

Zoladz Method

Unlike the Karvonen method the Zoladz method determines 5 exercise zones which are calculated by subtracting "zone adjuster" values from your maximum heart rate and then offsetting by 5 in either direction. For example we'll use 5 zone adjuster values.

Target Heart Rate Zone = Maximum Heart Rate – Zone Adjuster (+ 5) and (-5)

Zone Adjuster 1 = 50 bpm (Easy Exercise)
Zone Adjuster 2 = 40 bpm
Zone Adjuster 3 = 30 bpm
Zone Adjuster 4 = 20 bpm
Zone Adjuster 5 = 10 bpm (Hard Exercise)

Continuing our example:

Target Heart Rate Zone 1 = (180 – 50) = 130, Zone 1 = 125 to 135
Target Heart Rate Zone 1 = (180 – 40) = 140, Zone 2 = 135 to 145
Target Heart Rate Zone 1 = (180 – 30) = 150, Zone 3 = 145 to 155
Target Heart Rate Zone 1 = (180 – 20) = 160, Zone 4 = 155 to 165
Target Heart Rate Zone 1 = (180 – 10) = 170, Zone 5 = 165 to 175

Alternative Method

This method is calculated as a percentage of your Heart Rate Reserve and is very similar to the Karvonen Method. The difference is that the Alternative Method seeks to create a set of useful training zones by assigning easy to understand labels to each of the zones rather than just a set of numbers and percentages. The formulas used to determine the zones are:

Fat Burning Zone Low = ((Heart Rate Reserve) x 0.50) + Resting Heart Rate
Fat Burning Zone High = ((Heart Rate Reserve) x 0.75) + Resting Heart Rate

Fitness Zone Low = ((Heart Rate Reserve) x 0.75) + Resting Heart Rate
Fitness Zone High = ((Heart Rate Reserve) x 0.85) + Resting Heart Rate

Continuing our example:

Fat Burning Zone Low = (106 x 0.50) + 74 = 127 bpm
Fat Burning Zone High = (106 x 0.75) + 74 = 154 bpm

Fitness Zone Low = (106 x 0.75) + 74 = 154 bpm
Fitness Zone High = (106 x 0.85) + 74 = 164 bpm

Moving beyond these zones is not recommended unless you are

working to improve athletic performance. Nonetheless, I will include these formulas for your reference.

Aerobic-Anaerobic Threshold Low = ((HR Reserve) x 0.85) + Resting HR
Aerobic-Anaerobic Threshold High = ((HR Reserve) x 0.90) + Resting HR

Finally, the zone which ranges from 90 to 100% of your Maximum Heart Rate represents all out effort and like the Aerobic-Anaerobic Threshold Zone above it is not recommended, but is included for your reference.

Anaerobic Training Zone Low = ((HR Reserve) x 0.90) + Resting HR
Anaerobic Training Zone High = Maximum Heart Rate

Clear as mud!?

Don't fret. I realize this can be a bit confusing, so I've created a table in the **Appendix** to help you find your Target Heart Rate Zones based on the Alternative Method above.

Chapter 3

"I'll have a double cheeseburger and an ice water."

The secrets to my success

Eating is essential to sustaining life and incidentally it is also one of the most enjoyable sensations we can experience. When I think of the top 5 things I couldn't live without (no pun intended), the top 5 things that bring joy to my senses, apart from the obvious necessity of it, eating tops the list.

Unfortunately, eating incorrectly can and did have the opposite effect on my healthy happy self.

Obviously we all have to eat and we all have our preferences of dining experiences and tastes. I'm fortunate to live in an area where the economy is primarily driven by tourism and as a result the restaurant industry is flourishing.

Driving to work, which is a relatively short 15 minute commute, I pass nearly a hundred restaurants of various cuisine. From mom-and-pop pancake cabins to convenience store grills to national fast food chains to Five Star dining establishments I pass by many, many restaurants which are sure to please the most finicky of pallets.

I said that I'm fortunate to live here and now that I know how to eat appropriately I truly am fortunate, but prior to my prehypertension diagnosis I wasn't so fortunate. I mean although I was at that time surrounded by restaurants such as I am today I didn't know how to eat appropriately.

For me it was and still is a struggle to eat properly.

I love hamburgers and I've made it sort of a personal quest to find the best burger in America. Well, I haven't really traveled abroad, so I suppose for now I'll concede to confining my quest to the southeast.

While I've had some awesome sit-down restaurant burgers made from choice cuts of ground steak, I don't really count those as true hamburgers. All things considered Hardee's has the best selection of mouth watering juicy 5 pound burgers at a single stop and Five Guys Burgers and Fries have a huge selection toppings for their nearly perfect patties, but I've not yet found a burger that can compete with the flavor combination of the iconic Burger King Whopper. Additionally, I've had some exceptionally tasty burgers from a couple of convenience store grills here in the foothills of the Smoky Mountains of Tennessee. And one of fondest childhood memories is savoring the delectable flavors dripping from a freshly made burger hot off the grill at Ramon-Coleman's General Store in Piney Virginia!

OK, sorry to go off on that tangent.

On top of my burger quest sweets and junk food were staples of my daily menu. Chocolate chip cookies, Oreos, ice cream drowned in gallons of hot fudge, and greasy potato chips found their way into my lunch box and onto my lap as I vegged out in front of the television. To make matters worse I was partaking of these tasty treats in the late hours of the evening and night.

Speaking of late evening and night snacking, how often do you get hungry for a snack and opt to reach for the easily accessible cookie jar and engulf half a dozen cookies before your hand leaves the jar? That was me too!

"Food Product"

Have you ever picked up a package of "cheese" slices in the grocery aisle and on the packaging read "processed cheese product?" Cheese product? Not cheese food? Well a lot of the things we eat shouldn't be considered food, but rather products. We may as well be eating the wrapper the product was packaged in since the nutritional benefits would be about the same...possibly less harmful?

I was eating a ton of refined flour and refined sugar food products. White sandwich bread and donuts were products I didn't think I could live without. However, when I began to understand the way our bodies process these refined flours and sugars and the potential they represent not only for obesity, but for diabetes and heart disease, and even depression and cancer, it was much easier for me to change my eating habits.

The first thing I did was replace the white sandwich bread with a variety of whole grain breads. Some are tastier than others, but overall I enjoy the flavor of most whole grain breads.

Additionally, I was eating two sandwiches everyday for lunch along with a bag of chips and some sort of snack cake. So I cut back to one sandwich and replaced the chips and snack cake with healthier alternatives such as fruit or a sandwich bag filled with dry breakfast cereal. And here I allowed myself to splurge a little and would fill my sandwich bag with sweetened cereals such as fruit hoops or honey nut o's.

The mention of snack cakes is a nice segue into another area that I desperately needed to change. As I said previously, I love to eat and one of my favorite ways to unwind at the end of the day was to relax in front of the television with a piece of chocolate cake, or a bowl of ice cream, or a stack of cookies and a glass of milk. So not only was I ingesting a ton of unhealthy calories, but I was doing it late at night which didn't give my body enough time to burn them off. If I had continued down that road of glutenous indulgence who knows where my health would be today?

Sadly, even though I knew those eating choices were unhealthy and could bring some severe consequences it wasn't until I was truly motivated to make a change that I decided to do something about it.

Here are a few things that I did to change my poor eating habits. I stopped the late evening and late night snacking on unhealthy food products. I replaced refined flour products with whole grain alternatives. I replaced whole and 2% milk with 1% and skim milk. And when I had a craving for a piece of chocolate cake I chose a piece from the middle which contained less icing than a piece from the side or corner.

In addition to these changes, I cut back on my portion sizes at meals. At first this was very difficult, because I was used to over eating and I didn't feel like I was getting full. But eventually my body adjusted and I soon realized that I didn't need to feel FULL, but rather I just needed to feel "not hungry" which could be achieved with a lot less food. In fact for dinner a majority of the time I'd have a bowl of cereal. Usually, a bowl of raisin bran or other whole grain cold high fiber cereal that helps me feel full.

And speaking of cereal lets segue once more before I reveal the dietary secrets to my success.

When we think of cereal we think of breakfast and on that note I want to stress the importance of eating breakfast. In today's fast paced society we often find it easier to skip breakfast rather than risking being late for school or work. However, it is extremely important to eat something for breakfast to get your metabolism going for the day.

I'm not a morning person and getting up early to cook a large breakfast just isn't going to happen. So it is much easier for me to grab a couple toaster pastries or a danish or a cinnamon roll and eat it at my desk when I get to work.

Regardless of what you choose to eat as long as you aren't over indulging on icing covered sweet rolls, eat something. Since I had made the other changes to my dietary habits I didn't feel that a not-so-healthy small breakfast would cause too much of a negative effect on my progress. So if you aren't able to have a large sit down breakfast consisting of eggs and fruits and whole foods and grains, a smaller not-so-healthy Pop Tart or danish might be OK. Just be sure to monitor your own personal progress and adjust your menu to your specific needs.

Sample Daily Menu

Breakfast	A couple toaster pastries or a danish or cinnamon roll. Cup of Coffee. *Glass of Water.
Lunch	Sandwich on whole grain bread. Fruit such as an apple or banana. Small bag of dry cereal in place of greasy high carb potato chips. (limit your consumption of potatoes as much as possible) Glass of Water.
Snack	Cereal bar with oats or granola or other whole grain. There are several bars that are very tasty that I eat without feeling guilty. Some are even covered in chocolate! Or Fruit. Or Nuts.
Dinner	Bowl of whole grain high fiber cold cereal with 1% milk. OR (if you want a full meal) Chicken breast cooked in barbeque sauce. Bowl of beans (pinto beans are my favorite) Chopped spinach or greens with vinegar. Glass of Water.
Late Snack	Serving of blueberries or grapes Handful of nuts (cashews, almonds, etc.) Small glass of grapefruit juice (no sugar or sweetener added)

*Drink water continuously throughout the day.

"The Secrets To My Success"

In addition to eating properly structured and scheduled meals I'd like to share with you a few tricks that have helped me along my journey. I said tricks, but they are really more like rules or guidelines that you may want to tattoo onto the backside of your hand so you don't forget them and so they will be uncomfortably in your face when you are tempted to cheat!

1. This Offer Won't Last Long

We talked about motivation earlier and now I'd like to add a footnote to that discussion. Aside from the obvious health benefits of exchanging the flab for fab, nothing seems to motivate me more than seeing someone with a great physique. So my first tip is to find a picture or video of someone who has a body that you would like to look like and put it some place that you will look at it often.

Watching sporting events such as track and field, swimming, gymnastics, triathlons, cross-fit competitions, body building, and exercise shows. Even mainstream sporting events such as basketball and soccer games can be inspiring. But for me the #1 inspirational media has been...wait for it... infomercials for exercise programs or equipment.

Set your DVR to record a few infomercials that you find inspiring or that you've been considering purchasing (come on I know you've considered it, we all have) and when your vegging out on the couch flipping through the channels debating whether or not workout today, scroll over to your saved infomercial and see how long you stay sunken into the cushions.

2. Gentlemen Start Your Engines

Eat before you exercise to fire up your metabolism. Depending on the weather and the amount of time you will be exercising you will want to modify your portions accordingly, but I like to fuel my workouts with a choice of the following. Approximately 15 minutes before you exercise drink a few ounces of water, sports drink, or grapefruit juice (don't drink too much). And.

1. One or two whole grain cereal bars and a handful of blueberries.

OR

2. Peanut butter on one or two pieces of whole grain sandwich bread. Slice up a banana and add it to the sandwich for an extra boost of energy.

OR

3. Two or three handfuls of nuts and a banana or a couple handfuls of blueberries.

3. May I go to the bathroom please?

Although this might be one of the most difficult choice's you will make, the goal of this choice might be the easiest to achieve. So the next time you feed a handful of quarters into that soda machine press the water button instead of that syrup filled sugary soft drink. Drink water almost constantly. A good rule of thumb is to drink eight 8 ounce glasses of water a day or 64 ounces total, but I don't know that it is necessary to drink quite that much. However, it is important to keep your body hydrated throughout the day which will help you perform better when it comes time to exercise. Drinking throughout the day will also keep your stomach from being empty and help to prevent some of those urges to reach for the cookie jar throughout the day.

4. Late Night Snack

OK, I know some people will tell you that you're not supposed to eat after 7pm or 8pm and I don't recommend having dinner in the late evening or night hours, but I seem to stay hungry all the time. So when the urge to snack hits me I reach for a can of nuts, or grab a few handfuls of blueberries or strawberries or grapes, or I have a bowl of cereal.

Additionally, I'm going to go a step further and recommend that you eat a couple handfuls of blueberries and/or drink a small glass of grapefruit juice each night before you go to bed. Just be sure that the grapefruit juice is not a cocktail or ruby red which may have a combination of other juices and sweeteners. If you can stomach it stick to the bitter, able to strip paint off the wall, grapefruit juice. It may take some getting used to the flavor or lack there of, but you're not drinking any more than 8 ounces per serving so you'll get used to the taste.

5. I mean...um...I-mune it

In the early days of my exercise program research I came across several advertisements for a new super fruit that promised to melt away the pounds. Well I wasn't willing to shell out my hard earned cash for what may have been the latest fad, so I researched this super fruit a little more. And my research actually uncovered some real benefits to including this strangely named fruit, the Acai berry, in my diet. Apparently, it is a great source of antioxidants and it helps to boost your immune system. So I felt that I really didn't have anything to lose by giving it a try. But instead of investing in a potential scam I decided to search my grocer's shelves for the fruit. Unfortunately, I couldn't find it in any form other juice and if I remember correctly it may have only been available mixed with pomegranate juice. However, as I continued my search I came across the berry in gelcap form being sold as a dietary supplement.

Eager to give it a try I purchased a couple bottles of the supplement and began taking the gelcaps daily as directed on the label. Now I don't really know if the pills aided my weight-loss since I had made so many changes to my lifestyle, but I continue to take them daily. If nothing else they are fueling my immune system with antioxidants.

6. Launch the Spuds

While the potato has been hailed as a super food throughout the ages, a recent study by Harvard University researchers has shown this super tuber to be a major contributor to the growing problem of obesity. I'm guessing that the preparation techniques and added ingredients had some bearing on those results, but I think another factor that needs to be considered is that our children are becoming more and more inactive. At any rate, you can't go wrong by eliminating or at the very least limiting the amount of fried versions of potatoes that find their way onto your plate. If you pack your lunch and worry that you won't find your lunch filling enough without that bag of potato chips, replace the chips with a bag of your favorite dry cereal. Obviously whole grain cereals are going to provide the most benefits, but without milk that sounds about as appetizing as munching on a piece of cardboard. So I would recommend a lightly sweetened cereal such as Honey Nut Cheerios®.

7. Slower is better

We live in a fast paced society. One in which immediate gratification has become the norm. We grab a cereal bar or toaster pastry as we head out the door in the morning on our way to work. We drive through the pickup window of a fast food restaurant for lunch and have most of it eaten by the time we pull back into the parking lot. We have access at the touch of a button to events happening half way around the world, as they are happening!

It is quite remarkable how quickly technology is developing and changing the way we live our lives. And although we haven't yet made it on par with the Jetsons if you pop in a movie from around 30 years ago, a film that attempted to represent the technology of the future, it's easy to see that we've surpassed even our own far fetched ideas of what life would be like in 2011. Unfortunately, along with these fantastic developments some not so fantastic ones have also followed suit. Chances are, since you are reading this book, you've also fallen prey to at least a nibble from the jaws of this beast we call obesity.

This monster is devouring our population and bringing with it disease and depression. It has laid hold of both young and old, rich and poor. It shows no prejudice and is a force to be reckoned with. However, as the popularity of such shows as The Biggest Loser are yet another indicator of the monster's lurking presence, they also prove that it is not invincible. There is hope and one thing we can do to calm the beast is simply slow down and not feed it with our frantic lifestyle choices.

Studies have shown that it takes approximately 10 to 20 minutes before the sensors in the stomach and digestive system signal the brain and tell it, "Hey we've got food!" Wow, 20 minutes to our fast paced trained bodies is an eternity. I mean in the 5 minutes it takes you to drive back to work during your lunch break you can probably eat a burger and polish it off with an order of fries and a large chocolate shake. So what do you do with the remaining 15 minutes. Most of us will reach for a cookie or order a hot fudge sundae because we "think" we are still hungry. The reality is we've already eaten more than enough, but haven't allowed enough time for the food to settle, so to speak.

Therefore, my 7th and final secret is to simply slow down. Take your time and enjoy the flavors of that burger. Remove the lid from your chocolate shake and scoop some out with your fries. Instead of hurrying through your meal, slow down and enjoy it! You'll eat less. You'll feel better. And you'll be well on your way to achieving your goals in record time.

Chapter 4

"If you build it, results will come."

The Original Backpack Gym

Since the purpose of this book is to help you get fit as quickly as possible I don't want to waist your valuable time with a lengthy introduction. Instead I'm going to get right to the point and move quickly to constructing the Barstool Body Backpack Gym.

As a teenager I spent a lot of time exercising with traditional home gym equipment. In my parents' basement I had a weight bench fully equipped with free weights, a straight bar, a curling bar, dumb bells, and leg curling machine. I also had a larger machine that used heavy duty resistance bands and it even had a butterfly chest machine.

While these machines and equipment were effective they also took up a lot of space. In my parents' basement space wasn't really an issue, but when I moved out from under my parents' roof and into my own place space was no longer a luxury. That's when the idea for a compact home gym came to me.

I realize that I could have gotten around the necessity for more space by joining my local gym and in fact that's exactly what I did.

At first it was great. The gym was equipped with every machine imaginable and I could work muscles most of us don't even have! Unfortunately, after the initial excitement wore off I found myself going to the gym less and less. And as my family began to grow and the responsibilities of being a husband and father were weighing on me it became increasingly difficult to fit time for exercise into my daily routine. So I went looking for a solution that would allow me to exercise at home.

I tried several options including an interesting "door-gym" which was a device made of a set of pulleys that attached to the top and bottom of a door. Long resistance bands with loops on each end were stretched between the pulleys and you connected handles through the looped ends of the resistance bands which allowed you to perform several exercises. This was my favorite of the devices I tested and it was really quite clever, but its one limitation was the

32

resistance bands couldn't provide enough resistance to be very effective.

Additionally, I found a few devices that were exceptional for a few specific exercises, but were limited to working only those specific groups of muscles for which they were designed.

As I continued to search for the perfect compact gym I soon realized that a complete all-in-one machine didn't exist. And among the devices that did work well there were a few muscle groups that were being overlooked altogether.

"Barstool Body Backpack Gym"

Then it hit me. Instead of trying to find a single machine that works every muscle group why not use the devices that work the individual muscle groups best. And then combine them to form the ultimate compact home gym. Thus the idea for the Barstool Body Backpack Gym was conceived.

As you will soon see the Backpack Gym isn't necessarily a device that can be handled as a single entity, but rather it is a concept comprised of exercise and non-exercise equipment complementing each other in such a way as to construct the ultimate home gym for compact spaces. Optimal effectiveness of the Backpack Gym requires that some of the components of the gym be utilized for additional functions beyond those for which they were initially designed. We'll talk more about this later when I introduce the *Invisible Home Gym.*

Throughout the book I layout the various components of the gym and walk you through the steps to construct the gym. And in the next few pages I show you how to construct the lateral pull down, chest fly crossover, and pullup training components of the gym.

The Components of the Gym

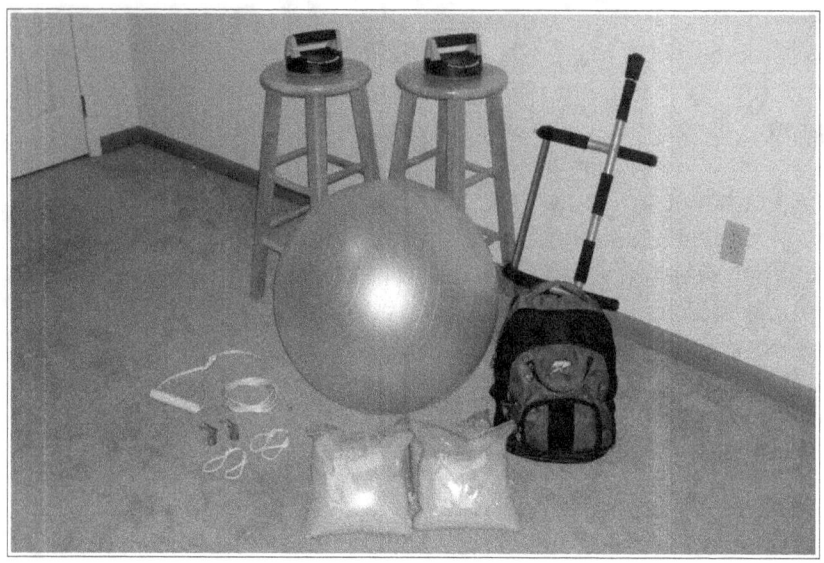

At first glance this hodgepodge of components looks more like a pile of stuff you might dump out of your storage closet. But believe it or not these items are all of the necessary components for the construction of the Backpack Gym.

Component Checklist

1. **Backpack.** Select the largest, sturdiest backpack you can find. You probably already have one that will work just fine. I used one of my kid's old backpacks. Just ensure the handle and straps are strong and the material wont tear or rip easily.

2. **Ziploc bags.** I chose to use gallon sized freezer bags, but you might want to get a couple different sizes.

3. **Sand.** Pick up a 50 pound bag of sandbox/playground sand from your local hardware store.

4. **Rope.** A length of rope approximately 25 feet should be

sufficient. Make sure it is rated to support at least 50 to 100 pounds depending on the amount of weight you use.

5. **Two Chain Spring Snap Links.** These should be able to support at least 50 to 100 pounds depending on how much weight you use.

6. **Two Pulleys.** These should be rated to support 50 to 100 pounds minimum depending on how much weight you use. Make sure there is little to no space between the pulley wheel and the wall of the pulley housing. The wheel should spin freely but not move side to side or wobble on the axle. If there is any space between the wheel and the pulley housing the rope could get jammed between the pulley wheel and pulley housing. It's a good idea to test the rope with the pulley while at the hardware store.

7. **Piece of 1" or 3/4" PVC pipe**. All you need is a length of PVC pipe about 8 inches long or a couple inches wider than your hand when grasping it in your fist.

8. **Pullup bar.** I chose one that allows for multiple hand positions, but a simple straight bar capable of supporting your body weight plus the amount of weight you might add to your workouts as described in the following chapters should work just fine.

9. **Two barstools.** Standard height barstools approximately 29 to 33 inches will work the best. My recommendation would be the tallest you can find that won't tip over easily.

10. **Rotating pushup handles.** Be sure to purchase a pair that have a good non-slip base. You'll see why this is important soon.

11. **Large exercise ball.** You can substitute a soft mattress for the exercise ball for the beginner's course, so this isn't necessary immediately.

Assemble the Components

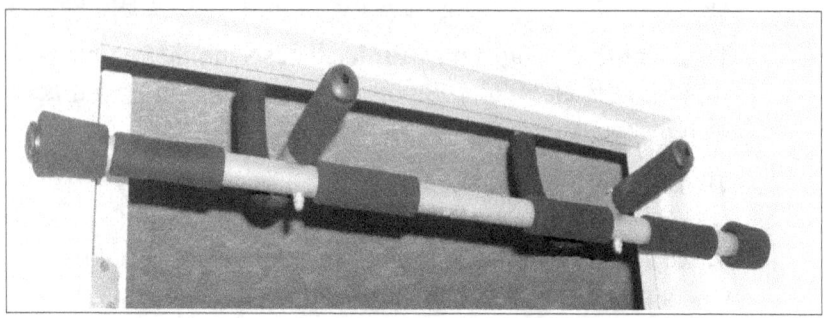

1. The first step is to mount your pullup bar according to the manufacturer's instructions. Since I live in a small 2 bedroom apartment I opted for a multiple position pullup bar that hangs from the trim around my door frame and utilizes leverage to stay in place. Your pullup bar may require you to screw brackets into your door frame. Whatever the case may be it is extremely important to follow the manufacturers instructions and test it thoroughly for strength and support before attempting any exercises.

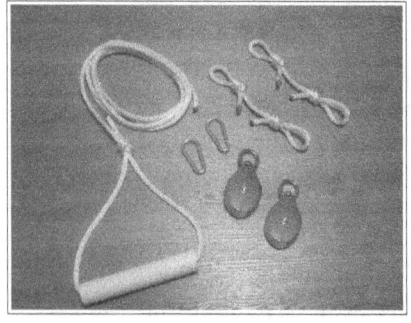 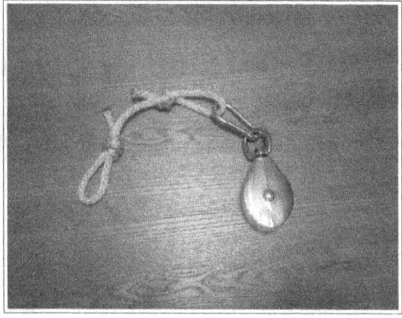

2. Cut two 1 foot sections of rope and tie both ends of each section into non-slipping loop knots so that you have two double-loop sections approximately 6 inches long each. Take the remaining length of rope and feed it through the 8 inch piece of PVC pipe and tie it off so that you have a large non-slipping loop knot with the PVC pipe inside the loop forming a handle.

3. Attach the Chain Spring Snap Links to the pulleys and connect one end of the double-loop rope section onto the chain spring snap link. You should have two complete units made up of one pulley, one chain spring snap link, and one double-loop rope section as pictured above.

Back, Triceps, Shoulders, and Chest

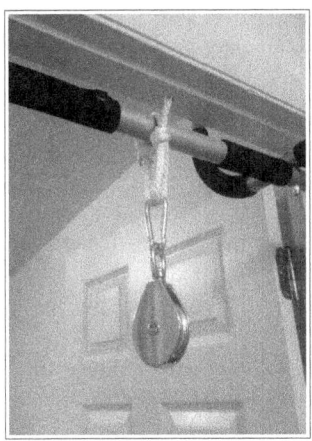

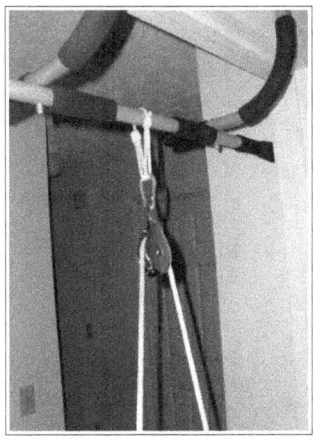

4. Hang the pulley from the pullup bar by wrapping one of the double-loop rope sections around the pullup bar and connect the Chain Spring Snap Link through the end loops.

5. Feed the free end of the length of rope you created in Step 2 above with the PVC pipe handle through the hanging pulley.

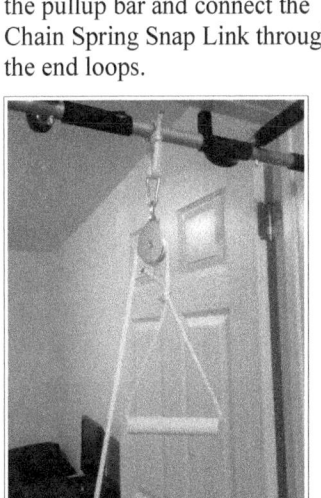

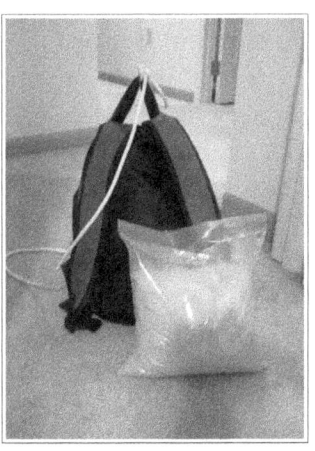

6. Pull the rope through the pulley so that the knot of the PVC handle loop touches the pulley.

7. Insert slide lock bags filled with sand into the backpack to achieve the amount of weight you require.* Tie the rope to the backpack handle or straps.

Pullup Training/Cable Crossover Machine

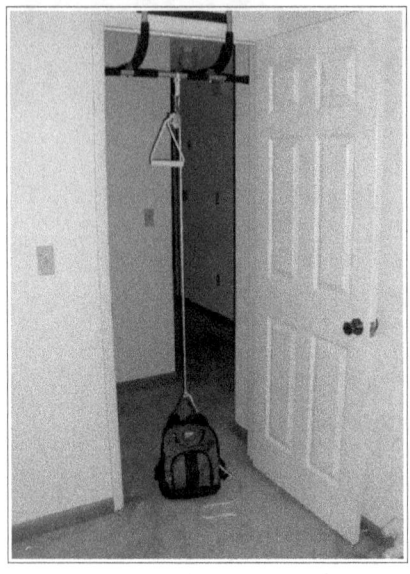

8. The completed Pullup Training and Cable Crossover Machine. Be sure to test the strength of the machine each time you assemble it by pulling down on the handle and lifting the backpack slightly off the floor. As pictured to the left, if you choose to use a pullup bar that is not fastened permanently to your door frame, make sure that when you pull on the handle you are pulling in the direction such that the leverage design of the pullup bar is engaged and being utilized. For instance in my example photo to the left, I pull down and towards the doorknob rather than away from the doorknob. Pulling away from the doorknob could cause the pullup bar to fall and potentially inflict injury or other damages.

* Fill as many slide lock bags with sand as you feel necessary to achieve a range of weights to use with the Backpack Gym. For each of my weights I filled a gallon sized freezer slide lock bag with sand, closed it, rotated it 90 degrees, and inserted it into another slide lock bag. This way I helped to ensure that if the slide lock bag opened it wouldn't leak sand all over my floor. This also gave me a double layer container which will help to prevent sand leaking if one of the bags is torn. Additionally, you might want to use a bead of super glue to seal the bags closed once you've filled them with sand.

"Look Mom, I tied my shoes."

Well maybe it isn't quite as exciting as first learning to tie your shoes, but it is VERY important to tie off the rope appropriately to the backpack so that it doesn't slip while you are exercising.

Follow these 5 steps to tie a simple knot that won't slip.

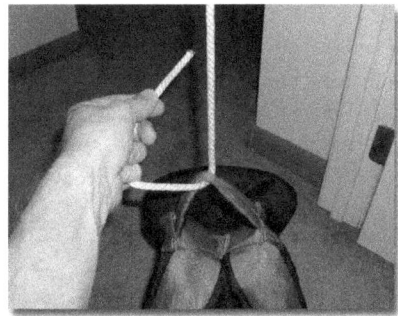

1. Thread the end of the rope through the top handle or through the shoulder straps of the backpack.

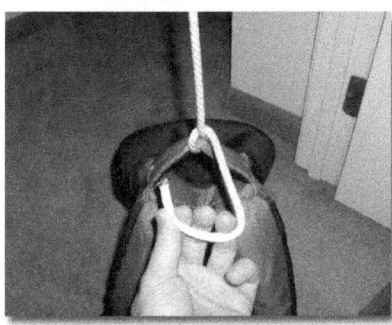

2. Take the end of the rope behind the hanging portion of the rope and pull it toward you.

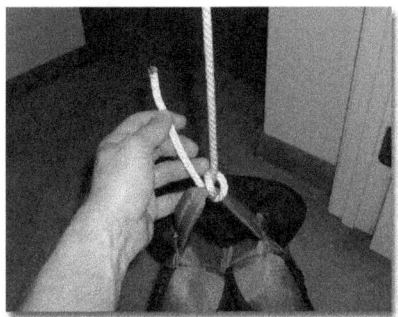

3. Push the end of the rope back under/through the top handle and pull it up and taught.

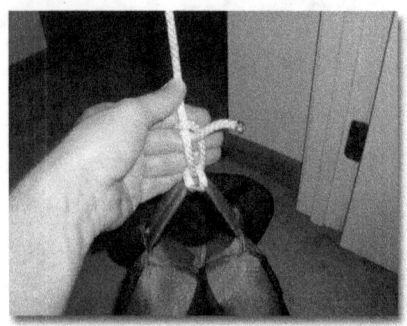

4. Hold the short end of the rope parallel to the right side of the hanging portion. Fold the short end at the half way point in a 90 degree angle pointing to the left so that the short end intersects in front of the hanging portion. Push the short end around the hanging rope and pull it back through the loop created to the right.

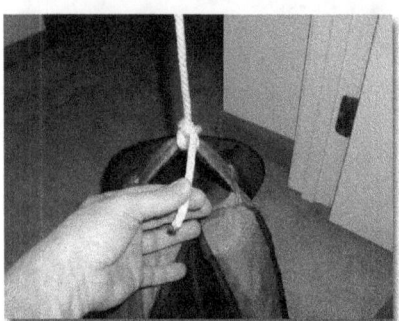

5. Pull the short end through the loop so that the knot is taught and will not slip. Be sure to test the strength of the knot and the backpack handle/straps by lifting the hanging portion of the rope.

"That was easy, but..."

So we've assembled the basic Backpack Gym, but you still have another pulley with its section of double-loop connector rope and a thousand extra feet of rope! And what about the barstools? We'll get to the second pulley and extra length of rope a little bit later, but concerning the barstools, here's something for you to try.

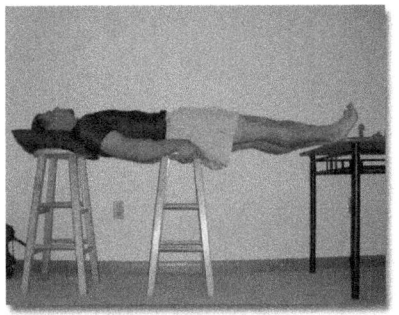 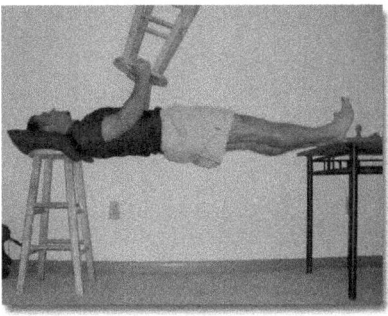

1. Most importantly, place a nice soft pillow on one of the barstools and position that barstool an appropriate distance from the table so that your heels will be supported on the table top while resting your head and upper portion of your shoulders on the pillow-topped barstool. You might find it easier to lay on the floor beside the barstools and table and adjust the position of the pillow-topped barstool while on the floor. Then take the second barstool and position it in between the barstool and the table and sit on it facing the table. Now rest your heels on the table and lay back onto the pillow-topped barstool. You're body should be perfectly (or very close to) straight.

2. Tighten your abdominal muscles, press your heels into the table and tighten your gluteal muscles (butt) so that your body is in a stiff reversed plank position as you stare at the ceiling. Now slowly remove the second barstool from underneath your backside and lift it over and around your torso so that the barstool in now upside down and supported by both of your hands. Pause for 10 to 15 seconds and continue the circular movement of the barstool down and around the opposite side of your torso and return it to the starting position under your backside. Repeat this motion for as many reps as you can until fatigued.

OK, if you can't do the above move, don't worry. I actually don't expect you to be able to at this point, but I simply wanted to present this as a mini-goal for you to work towards. And I have no doubt that you will be able to do it soon enough.

Chapter 5

"Barstools aren't just for sitting."

Invisible Home Gym

How many times have you sat on your barstool eating a piece of pie and sipping a creamy sugar filled cup of coffee. Or when was the last time you sat on that same barstool enjoying your favorite beverage while the only benefit the barstool provided was a comfortable perch. The thought of exercise at those particular moments was probably the farthest thing from your mind. Well, all of that is about to change and the next time you utilize a barstool to support your unhealthy indulgences, you won't be able to walk away from the barstool without thinking, "Hmm, I suppose I should do a few reps to burn off that pie."

"Barstool Body Invisible Home Gym"

Like the Backpack Gym the phrase Invisible Home Gym describes a concept rather than a particular device. "Invisible" refers to the idea of using equipment that wasn't designed for the purpose of exercise to create exercise equipment. For instance a major component of the Backpack Gym is a barstool which obviously wasn't designed to function as home gym equipment. However, in the following pages I will show you how to utilize one and two barstools to create such home gym equipment. Additionally, because I designed the gym for small spaces I wanted it to be as inconspicuous as possible. So when not in use most of the components can be stored in the backpack. Thus making it virtually invisible and extremely portable.

Let's continue constructing the Backpack Gym as we practice the concept of the Invisible Home Gym.

"Portable Gym"

One of the reasons I chose to use a backpack for my gym is that it would make an excellent storage container for the various components of the gym. However, when my pullup bar is completely assembled it is too large to fit into the backpack and disassembling it is impossible without the use of tools. So I made a very small modification to the out-of-box materials and now my pullup bar can be disassembled in a few seconds.

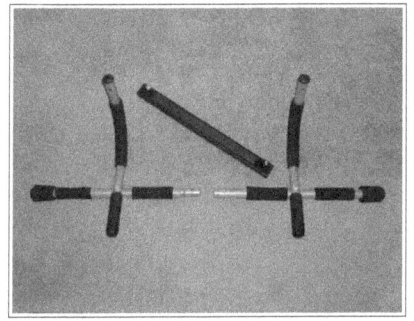

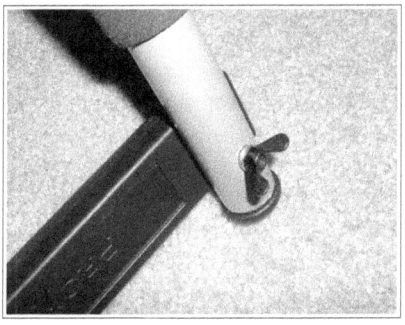

1. Fully assemble the pullup bar according to the manufacturer's instructions. Remove the plastic rectangular cross beam support.

2. Replace the manufacturer supplied nuts with finger tightening wing nuts and reassemble the plastic rectangular cross beam support. That's it! Told you it was a simple modification.

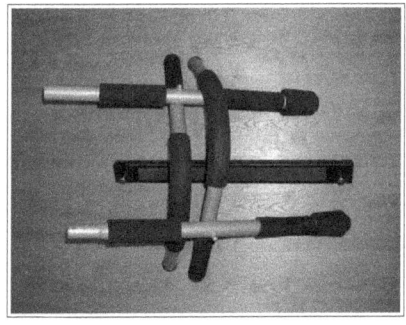

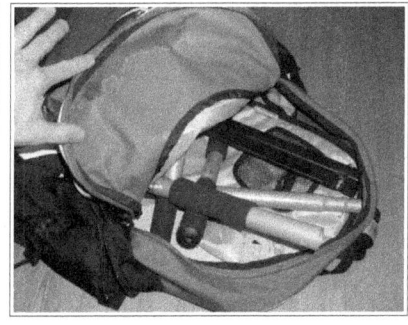

3. Disassemble the pullup bar.

4. Store the pullup bar and other gym components in the backpack.

*Please note that making this modification may void the manufacturer's warranty and should be done at your own risk.

Pullup Training, Dips, Leg Raises

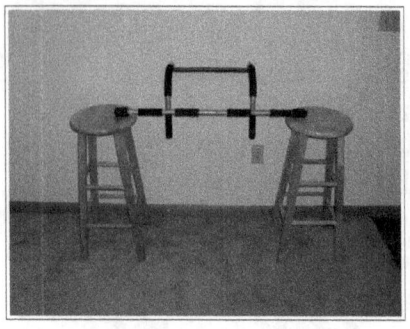 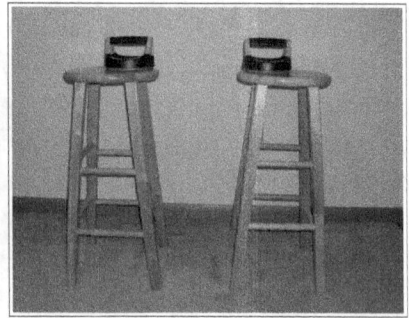

1. Place two barstools a few inches away from the wall and separate them with enough distance that you can rest your pullup bar or other strong pole across the barstools. A carpet floor works best.

2. Place two barstools slightly wider than your hips being careful not to place them too far apart. Set a rotating pushup handle on each barstool near the center, but not too close to the edge. A carpeted floor works best.

Biceps, Shoulders, Traps, and Back

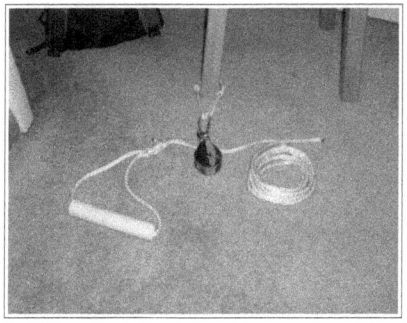

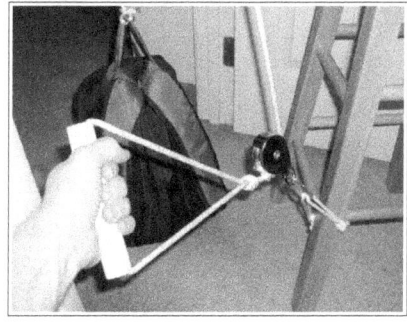

1. Hang one pulley from the pullup bar as you did for the Pullup Training and Cable Crossover Machine. Attach the other pulley around the base of one of the legs of your barstool.

2. Feed the free end of the PVC handle rope through the pulley and pull the slack all the way through so that the knot of the PVC handle loop touches the pulley.

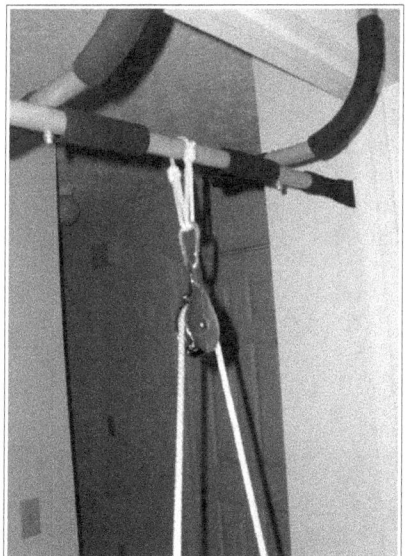

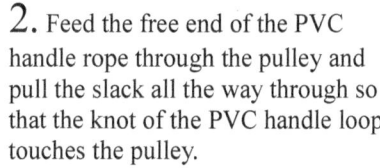

3. Feed the free end of the PVC handle rope through the hanging pulley and pull the slack all the way through.

4. Insert a number of sand bags into the backpack to achieve the amount of weight you require. Tie the rope to the backpack's top handle or straps.

Seated Curling/Lateral Raise Machine

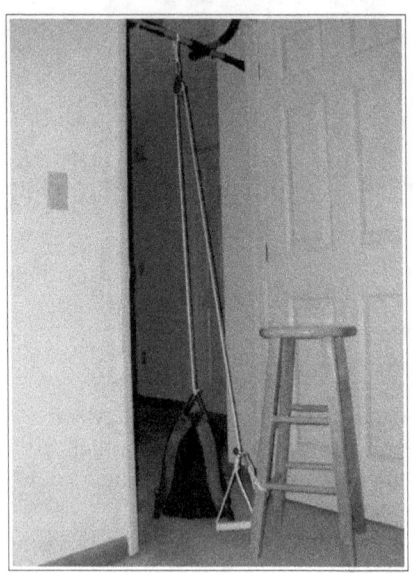

5. The completed Curling and Seated Lateral Raise Machine. Be sure to test the strength of the machine each time you assemble it. As pictured to the left if you choose to use a pullup bar that is not fastened permanently to your door frame make sure that you position your barstool in such a way that when you pull on the handle the tension on the rope is in the direction that engages the leverage design of the pullup bar. For instance in my example photo to the left I positioned my barstool inside the room in the direction that the door opens placing the barstool adjacent to the door. Positioning the barstool on the outside of the room would cause the tension on the rope to pull in the opposite direction and not engage the leverage design of the pullup bar which could cause the pullup bar to fall and potentially inflict injury or other damages.

Chapter 6

"Stoke the FIRE!"

Stop *spending* time on exercise.
Start *investing* time in a healthier happier you.

The primary benefit of incorporating strength training exercise into your weight-loss program is that you will be building lean muscle which in turn will boost your metabolism and help you to burn calories even when you're not exercising.

A traditional low calorie diet melts away the fat leaving you with a trimmed physique to which you might respond by inviting all of your buddies over for a celebration bonfire fueled by your old wardrobe. However, should you choose to replace the beans and rice with burgers and fries that bulge you defeated with the onslaught of low calorie meals is going to return with a vengeance and reclaim its previous territory. The reason for this is that lean muscle is an unfortunate casualty of the low-calorie-only battle.

I may be going out on a limb here, but I'm guessing your goal is to not only lose wait but to keep it off for good. If that is correct then it's imperative that you build lean muscle which boosts your metabolism and keeps the calorie burning fire roaring!

Now, don't get me wrong. As we discussed in the last chapter a change in your eating habits is most likely going to be necessary. But in addition to your low calorie meals you need to incorporate some cardiovascular exercise into your routine. So before you begin your strength training program which will fuel the flames you first need to kindle the fire, apply some spark, and get the fire burning.

When my journey began even though I could ride 20 miles on my road bike the thought of running a single mile was like fingernails on a chalkboard. Let me back up for a second. As I discussed cycling previously I feel that I might have come across a little too harshly towards the benefits of cycling, but that was not my intention at all. Quite the opposite. I'm a huge fan of cycling! In fact there are very few things that I enjoy more than a brisk ride through the rolling hills of East Tennessee. Cycling is one of the most enjoyable and effective "non-exercise" exercises you can perform and if you have the time to spend cycling I highly recommend it. However, since my goal was to achieve a healthier me as quickly as possible with minimal effort, the amount of time I needed to spend cycling wouldn't fit into my schedule. So I temporarily shelved my cycling shoes and replaced them with a pair of running shoes.

When I first began running it was very hard on my feet, shins, and legs. My feet hurt. My shins felt like I hit a growth spurt. My legs cramped. I felt like Frankenstein when I walked and I could barely sit down and stand up. But I stuck with it and eventually my body adjusted to the impact and new movements.

Running quickly became my cardiovascular exercise of choice. Why? It was simple. It didn't require any fancy equipment to maintain. It could be done indoors if the weather was bad. And perhaps most importantly, it provided an extremely effective cardiovascular workout in a fraction of the time it would have required me to achieve a similarly effective workout on my bicycle.

But how much time did I need to spend running for it to be effective? Again, I was trying to achieve noticeable results with minimal effort in the shortest amount of time possible and what I found was quite surprising.

I started out doing very short intervals of 5 to 10 minutes and worked up to 15 and 20 minute intervals. As my conditioning improved I was able to run for longer periods of time, but I didn't want spend longer than 15 to 20 minutes so I intentionally kept the majority of my sessions within these limits.

Combined with better dietary habits the cardio sessions formed a strong foundation upon which to build my Barstool Body Invisible Home Gym.

With the foundation formed we're now ready build the strength training portion of the Barstool Body Invisible Home Gym.

I realize that everyone reading this book isn't at the same fitness level and to accommodate I've attempted to split the exercise moves into two groups:

1. Beginner
2. Intermediate/Advanced

Since the majority of us are wanting to get rid of those pesky extra pounds around our midsections we'll begin with exercises that target the abdominal and oblique muscles.

Quick Tip

One of the simplest modifications you can do to improve the most famous of all abdominal exercises is to use a mattress to perform the abdominal crunch/situp. The mattress allows the contour of your upper and lower back and buttocks to stay in a more natural position than does lying on the floor. This takes the strain off of your lower back and aids the engagement of your target muscle groups. Additionally, if you slide you're feet slightly over the edge of the mattress you will get a better stretch between reps. And as your fitness level improves move the mattress onto the floor and position yourself so that you're sitting on the edge of the mattress with your feet pointing towards the middle of the mattress and lay back so that your shoulders rest on the floor. Then raise your shoulders off of the floor and perform a full situp. As a further challenge you might also attempt to keep the mattress elevated off the floor and position yourself so that you are sitting on the edge of the mattress the same as above. Then anchor your feet in such a way that you can lay backwards off the edge of the mattress lowering your shoulders and head as close to the floor as possible and return to a seated position. As this move can strain your lower back and is a potential cause for injury, please use caution before performing this move.

Chapter 7

"Gather the Logs"

Lay some planks and build the foundation

In the previous chapters we've discussed various concepts and assembled the equipment necessary to allow you to perform the exercises which utilize these concepts and equipment. Therefore, in the following chapters it is my goal to gather the remaining logs and stack them into easily accessible piles which will allow you to grab a piece of wood and toss it into the fire with minimal effort. Then sit back and enjoy the validating warmth of the flames as they burn through your body building lean muscle mass and melting away the fat.

This chapter focuses on developing the various exercise moves which add the finishing touches to the Barstool Body Invisible Home Gym. I've provided an explanation of how to effectively perform each movement along with images in which I've attempted to demonstrate proper form, although I'm sure you will look much better than I do as you perform the exercises. At the end of the chapter you will have a large inventory of exercises that you will then be able to plug into your very own exercise program.

The Plank Position

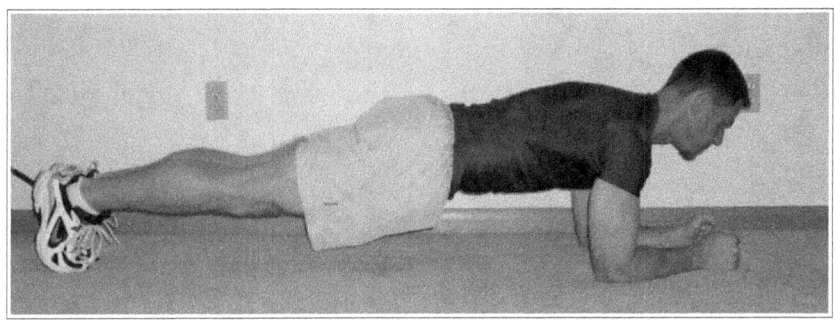

1a. The plank position is a very simple move, but can be a very effective move to strengthen your core when performed correctly. To perform the move lay on the floor face down and prop up on your elbows and forearms. Then straighten your legs and lift your knees off the floor making your body as straight as possible. Your body should now be suspended almost parallel to the floor supported by your toes, elbows, and forearms. Now engage your abdominal muscles by slightly rotating your pelvis toward the floor. Hold for 30 seconds to 1 minute.

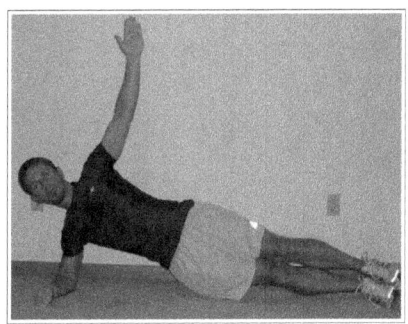

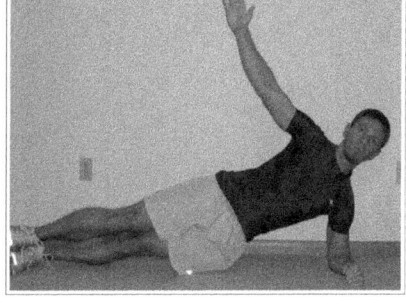

1b. From the plank position rotate your body so that you are resting on your right forearm and elbow, the side of your right foot, and your left shoulder is pointing toward the ceiling. Keep your spine, hips, and legs in a straight line and hold the position with your left hand extended toward the ceiling. Hold for 30 seconds to 1 minute.

1c. From the plank position rotate your body so that you are resting on your left forearm and elbow, the side of your left foot, and your right shoulder is pointing toward the ceiling. Keep your spine, hips, and legs in a straight line and hold the position with your right hand extended toward the ceiling. Hold for 30 seconds to 1 minute.

Ergonomic Mattress Crunches/Situps

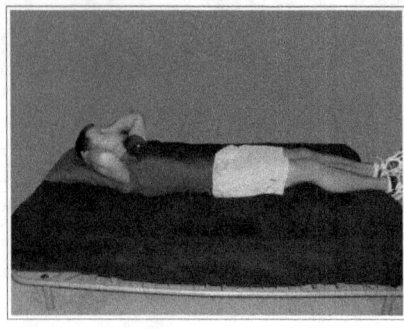 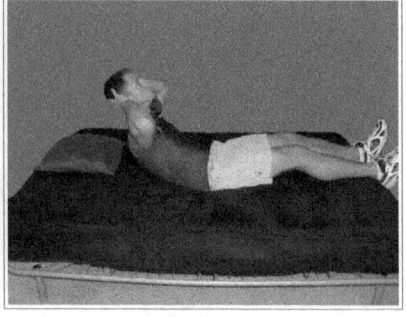

2a. Lay on a mattress with your feet slightly hanging over the edge. Rest your head on a pillow and place your hands on the sides of your head with your elbows pointing outward.

2b. Engage your abdominal muscles and lift your shoulders off the mattress to slightly more than 45 degrees (don't pull your head with your hands). Hold the position for 1 to 2 seconds and slowly lay back returning to the start position. That's 1 rep.

Ergonomic Mattress Twist Crunches/Situps

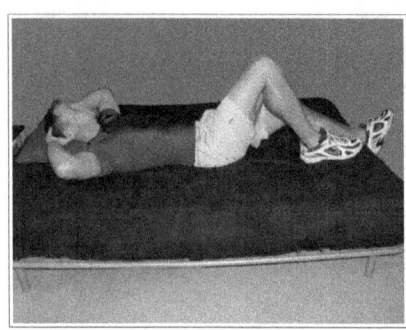 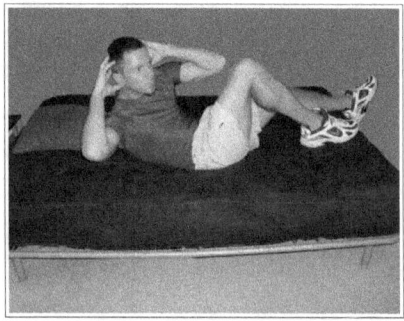

3a. Lay on a mattress with your left foot slightly hanging over the edge and your right foot pulled in so that your right knee is at a 90 degree angle pointing toward the ceiling. Rest your head on a pillow and place your hands on the sides of your head with your elbows pointing outward.

3b. Engage your abdominal and oblique muscles lifting your shoulders off the mattress and rotating your left elbow around to touch your right knee. Hold the position for 1 to 2 seconds and slowly lay back returning to the start position. That's 1 rep. Repeat the movement with your opposite knee and elbow.

Exercise Ball Crunches/Situps

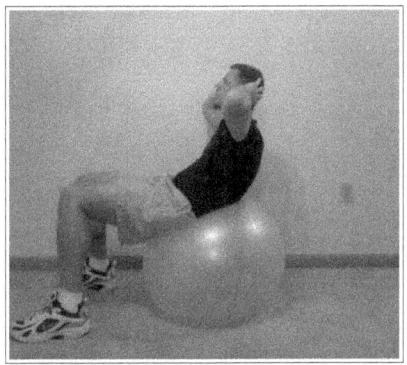 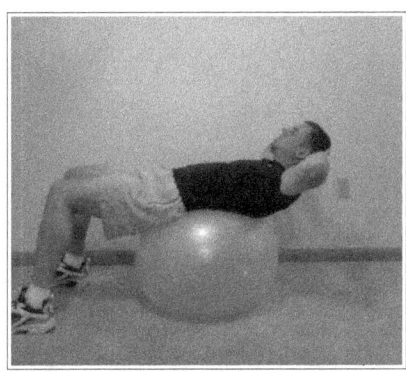

4a. Sit on top of the exercise ball with your feet flat on the floor, knees apart and bent at 90 degrees, and hands on the sides of your head. Move slightly forward so that the ball rolls into the curve of your lower back. Lean back slightly while engaging your abdominal muscles.

4b. Lay back lowering your shoulders toward the floor until your torso is in a straight line with your thighs. Now raise your shoulders while engaging your abdominal muscles as you return to the starting position (4a). Hold for 1 to 2 seconds. That's 1 rep.

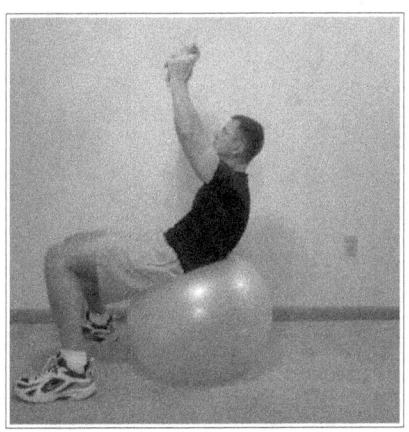 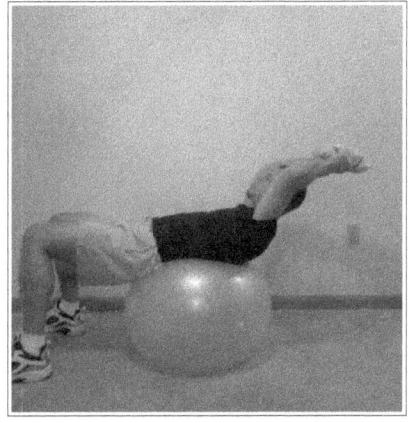

5a. Position yourself on the exercise ball as in 4a above, but instead of placing your hands on the sides of your head hold a sand bag above your head.

5b. Lay back lowering the sand bag toward the floor until your torso is in a straight line with your thighs. Raise the sand bag while engaging your abdominal muscles as you return to the starting position (5a). Hold for 1 to 2 seconds. That's 1 rep.

Leg Raises

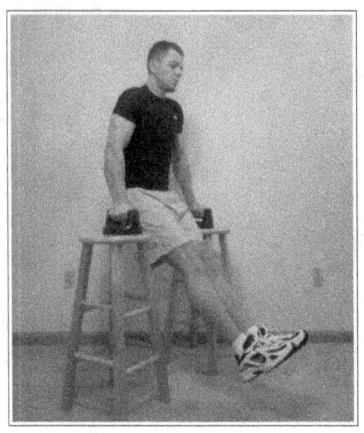 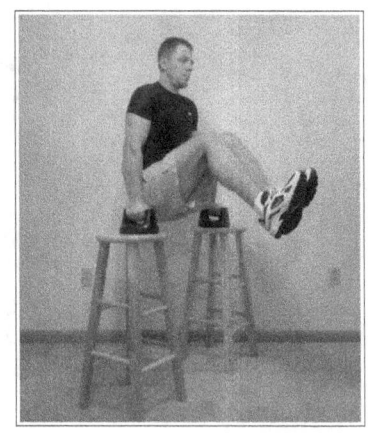

6a. Support yourself on the Leg Raise machine with your feet off the floor, legs straight, and at a 45 degree angle to the floor. Hold for 2 seconds.

6b. Raise your knees toward your chest and lower them slowly to the starting position. That's 1 rep.

Bicep Leg Raises

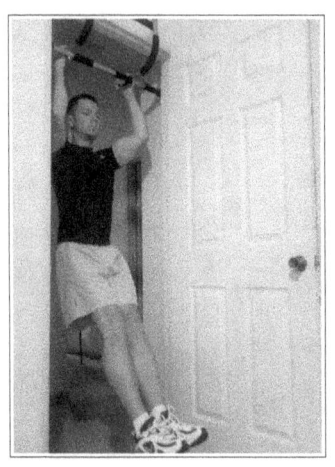 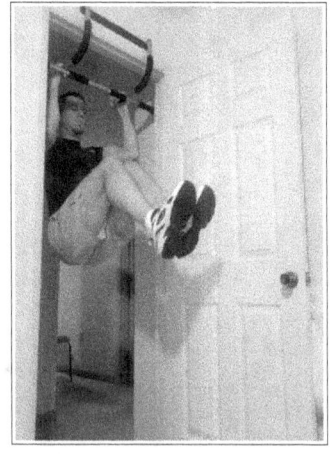

7a. Grasp the pullup bar and do a half pullup so that your elbows are bent at 90 degrees, your feet are off the floor, legs straight, and at a 45 degree angle to the floor. Hold for 2 seconds.

7b. While keeping your elbows bent raise your knees toward your chest and lower them slowly to the starting position. That's 1 rep.

Diamond Pushups

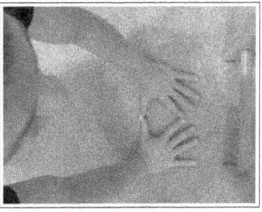 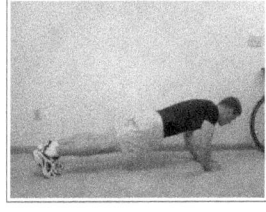 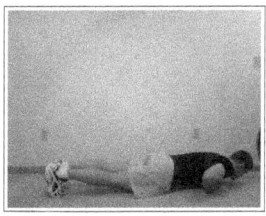

8a. Lay face down on the floor with your legs straight, feet together, and hands palm down and positioned under your shoulders. Engage your abdominal muscles by rotating your pelvis toward the floor and push up with your arms until they are almost straight. Slide your hands together so that the tips of your index fingers and thumbs touch.

8b. Keeping your abs flexed slowly lower your upper body to about an inch above your hands and hold for 3 seconds. Then push up as quickly as possible to the starting position.

Elevated Pushups

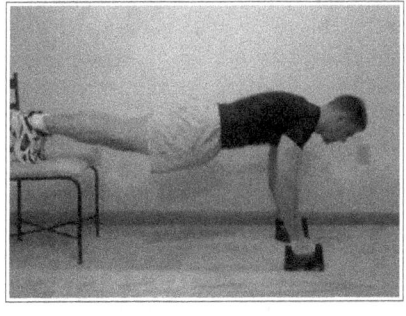 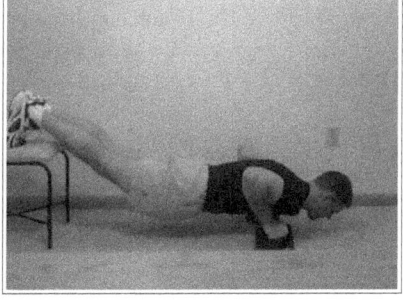

9a. Place rotating pushup handles shoulder width apart on the floor a short distance in front of your chair. Position yourself on your knees and grasp the pushup handles. Walk your feet backwards and up onto the chair and push up with your arms until your body is in a straight line and your elbows are slightly bent.

9b. Engage your abdominal muscles by rotating your pelvis slightly toward the floor. Slowly lower your upper body until your chest is 1 to 2 inches above the floor. Hold the position for 3 seconds and push up as quickly as possible to the starting position. That is 1 rep.

Weighted Elevated Pushups

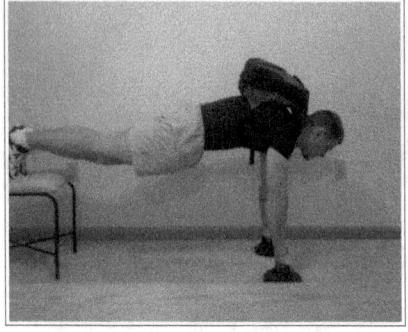 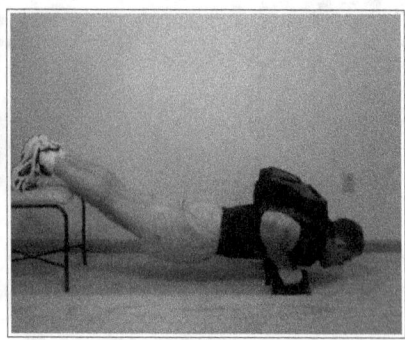

10a. Fill your backpack with an appropriate amount of sand bag weights and position it on your upper back approximately between your shoulder blades. Place rotating pushup handles shoulder width apart on the floor a short distance in front of your chair. Position yourself on your knees and grasp the pushup handles. Walk your feet backwards and up onto the chair and push up with your arms until your body is in a straight line and your elbows are slightly bent.

10b. Engage your abdominal muscles by rotating your pelvis slightly toward the floor. Slowly lower your upper body until your chest is 1 to 2 inches above the floor. Hold the position for 3 seconds and push up as quickly as possible to the starting position. That is 1 rep. Be careful to keep the backpack positioned on your upper back approximately between your shoulder blades.

Note: A set of pushups is defined as the number of reps you can perform until you break good form. So when you begin to arch your back or your knees begin to hinge and you are unable to keep your body in a straight line stop there marking the end of the current set.

Basic Dips

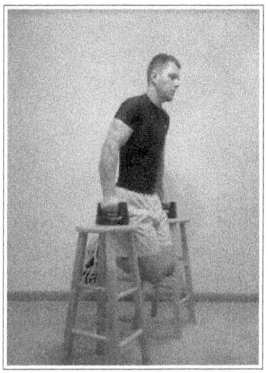 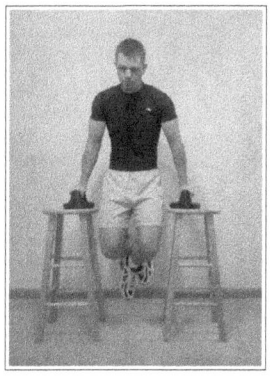 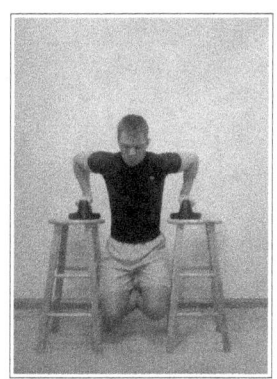

11a. Support yourself on the Leg Raise and Dip machine with your elbows slightly bent and your knees bent to approximately 90 degrees with your feet under your buttocks. Test the stability of the Leg Raise and Dip machine and adjust the positioning of the barstools and rotating pushup handles until the machine is stable. Placing the barstools on a carpeted floor works best. Also, use rotating pushup handles with non-slip bottoms.

11b. Focus on working your chest. Slowly lower your body until your shoulders are lower than your elbows. Pause then push up as quickly as possible to the starting position. That is 1 rep.

Abdominal Dips

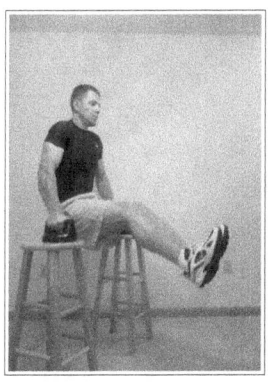 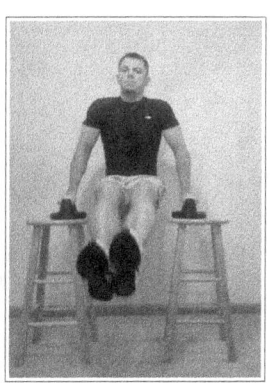 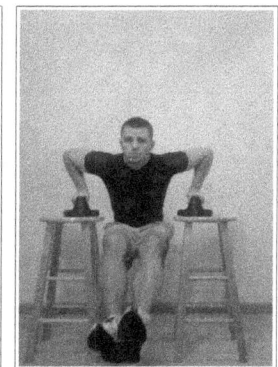

12a. Support yourself on the Leg Raise and Dip machine as in 11a above, but with your legs extended and parallel to the floor. Engage your abdominal muscles and keep them flexed throughout the entire movement.

12b. Perform the move as described in 11b above keeping your legs parallel to the floor and abs engaged.

Pullup Training

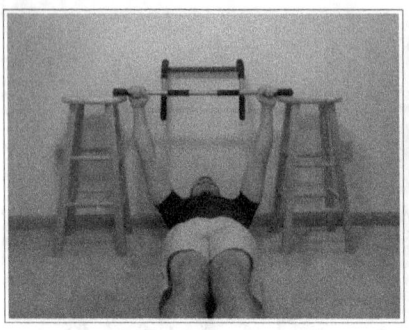 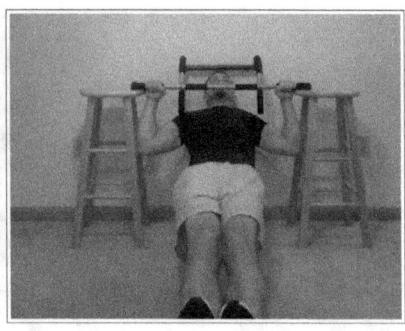

13a. Lay on your back and position yourself under the pullup training station between the two barstools. Grasp the pullup bar slightly wider than shoulder width. With your feet together, engage your abdominal muscles, and straighten your body.

13b. Keeping your body as straight as possible slowly pull your upper body up toward the pullup bar until your chin touches the bar. You should be pivoting on your the heels of your feet. Hold the position for 1 to 2 seconds and slowly return to the starting position. That is 1 rep.

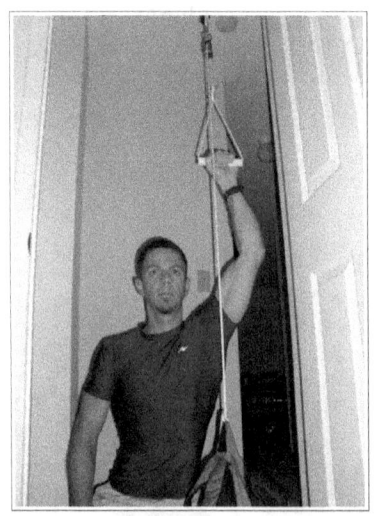 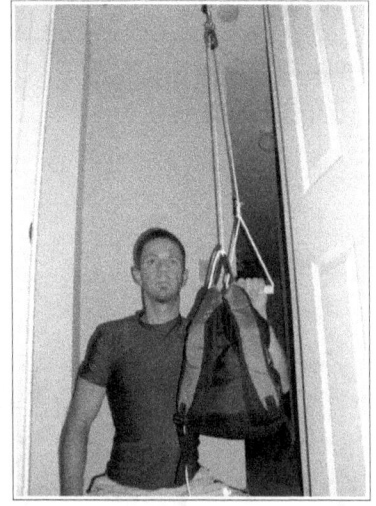

14a. Assemble the Pullup Training/Cable Crossover Machine and position yourself on the floor on your knees facing the machine. Grasp the PVC handle.

14b. Keeping your torso as straight as possible slowly pull down on the PVC handle until the handle touches your shoulder. Hold the position for 1 to 2 seconds and slowly return to the starting position. That is 1 rep.

Standard Wide Grip Pullups

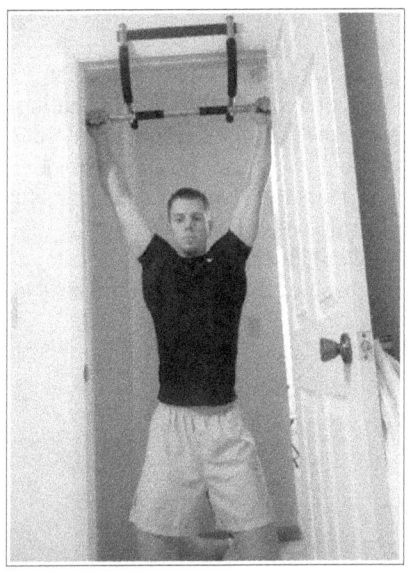

15a. Grasp the pullup bar with your palms facing away from you and your hands positioned wider than shoulder width so that the outside of your hands are lightly touching the inside of the door frame. Lift your feet behind you bending your knees to approximately 90 degrees.

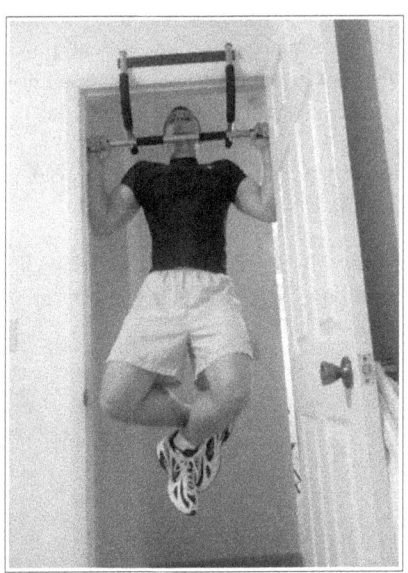

15b. Keeping your knees bent, pull yourself up as quickly as possible until your chin is slightly higher than the pullup bar. Pause briefly and slowly lower yourself to the starting position. That is 1 rep.

Note: When first starting a pullup regimen instead of returning all the way to the starting position you may find it easier to keep your elbows slightly bent at the bottom of each rep.

Weighted Wide Grip Pullups

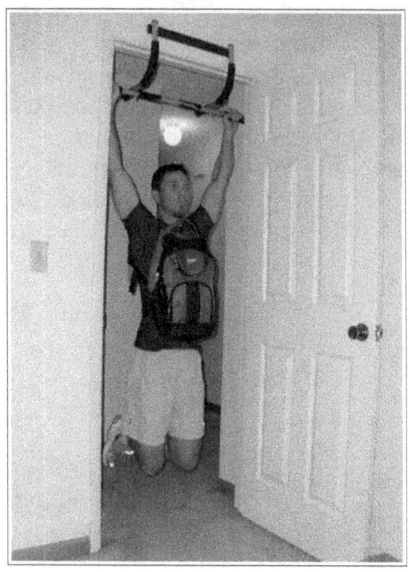

16a. Wearing the sandbag filled backpack in reverse (on your chest instead of your back) grasp the pullup bar with your palms facing away from you and your hands positioned wider than shoulder width so that the outside of your hands are lightly touching the inside of the door frame. Lift your feet behind you bending your knees to approximately 90 degrees.

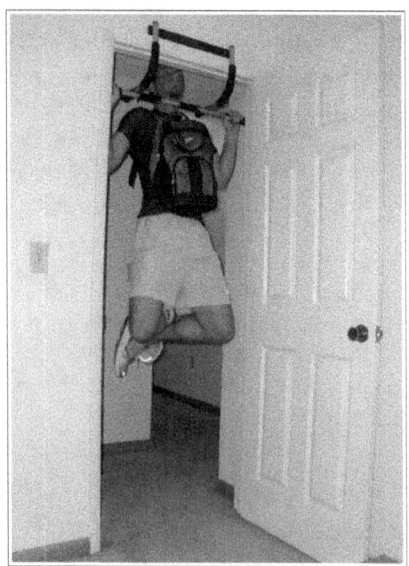

16b. Keeping your knees bent, pull yourself up as quickly as possible until your chin is slightly higher than the pullup bar. Pause briefly and slowly lower yourself to the starting position. That is 1 rep.

Note: Fill the backpack with enough sand bag weights so that you can do 8 to 10 reps max.

Abdominal Wide Grip Pullups

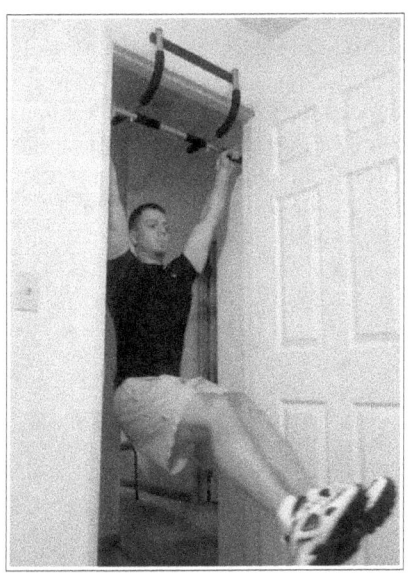

17a. Grasp the pullup bar as you did in exercise move 15a above, but with your legs extended in front of you and parallel to the floor. Engage your abdominal muscles and keep them flexed throughout the entire movement.

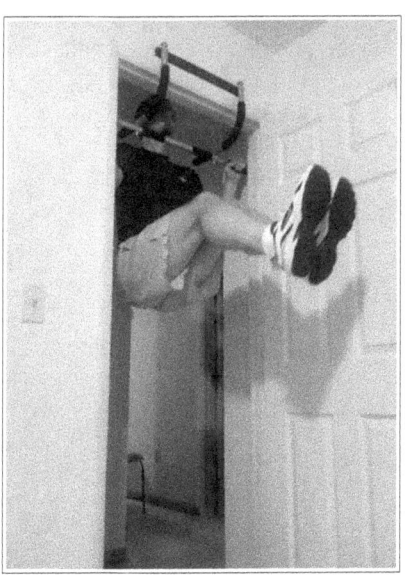

17b. Keeping your legs parallel to the floor and your abdominal muscles engaged pull yourself up as quickly as possible until your chin is slightly higher than the pullup bar. Pause briefly and slowly lower yourself to the starting position. That is 1 rep.

Note: When first starting a pullup regimen instead of returning all the way to the starting position you may find it easier to keep your elbows slightly bent at the bottom of each rep.

Extreme Abdominal Wide Grip Pullups

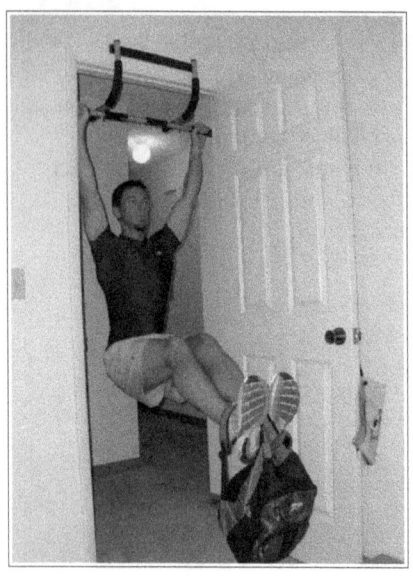

18a. Fill your backpack with 5 to 10 pounds of sand bag weights and step through the backpack's shoulder straps with one foot through each strap. Grasp the pullup bar with a wide grip and extend your legs in front of you until they are parallel to the floor.

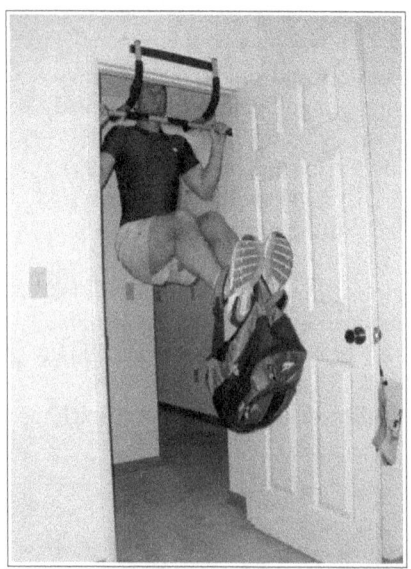

18b. Keeping your legs parallel to the floor pull yourself up as quickly as possible until your chin is slightly higher than the pullup bar. Pause briefly and slowly lower yourself to the starting position. That is 1 rep.

Cable Crossover Chest Flex

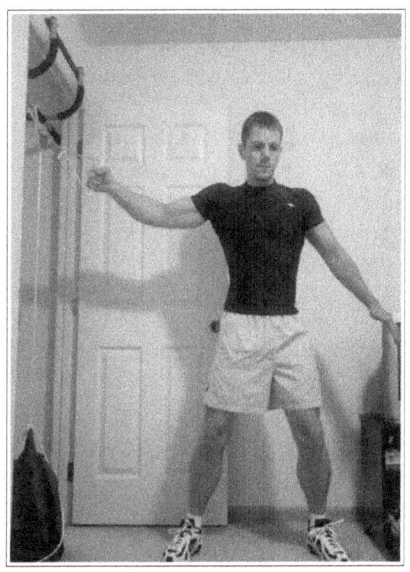

19a. Assemble the **Pullup Training/Cable Crossover Machine** . Grasp the PVC handle with your right hand and position yourself on the side of the machine so that when you pull on the PVC handle you engage the leverage design of the pullup bar. While holding the PVC handle move away from the machine so that your arm is extended to your side and elbow slightly bent. Position your feet shoulder width apart.

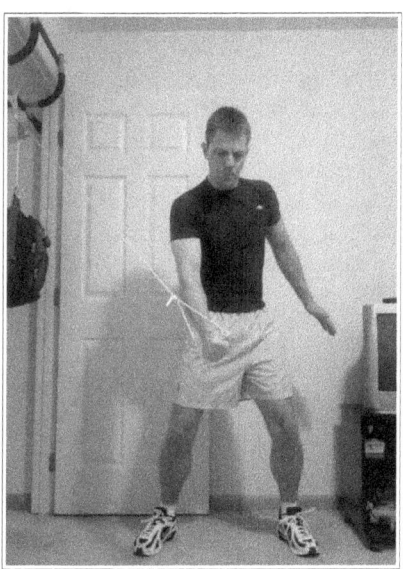

19b. Slowly pull the PVC handle across your torso down and in front of your waist. When your arm is straight out in front of you engage your abdominal muscles and slightly rotate your right shoulder down and to the left performing a standing twist crunch. Hold the position for 1 to 2 seconds and slowly return to the starting position. That is 1 rep.

Seated Lateral Raise

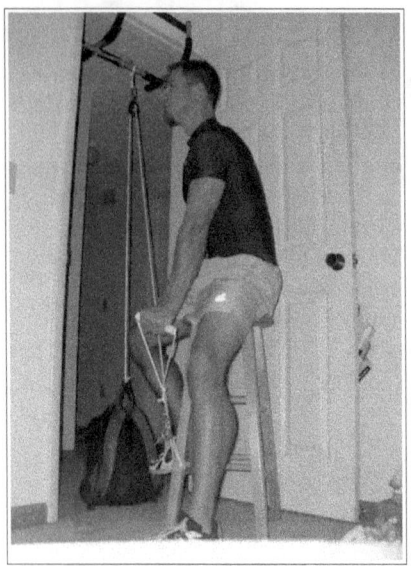

20a. Assemble the **Seated Curling/Lateral Raise Machine**. Remember to place the barstool on the side of your pullup bar so that the tension from the rope engages the leverage design of the pullup bar. Sit on the barstool with your legs straddling the pulley and PCV handle rope. Grasp the PVC handle with your palm face down. Keep your back straight and elbow slightly bent.

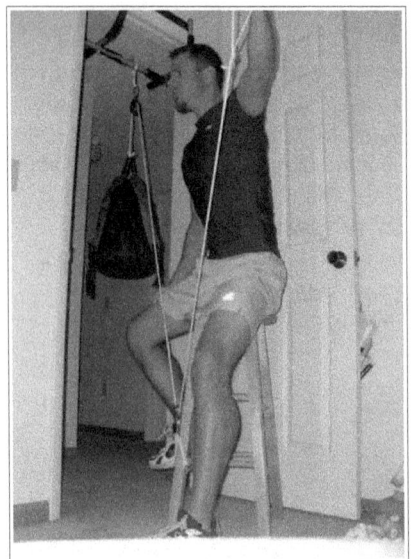

20b. With your back straight and elbow slightly bent lift your arm diagonally up and away from your body. Stop when your hand is over your head and your arm is at a slightly higher than 45 degree angle. Hold the position for 2 to 3 seconds and return to starting position. That is 1 rep.

Bicep Curls

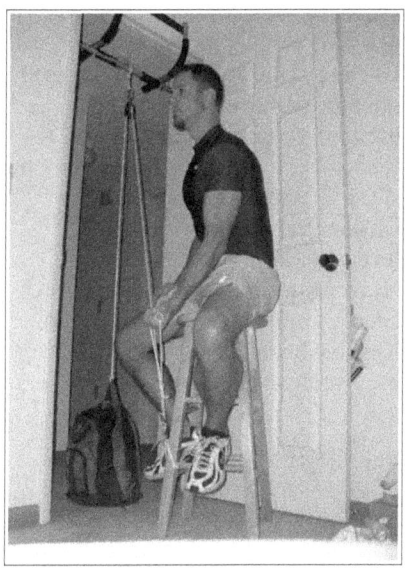

21a. Assemble the **Seated Curling/Lateral Raise Machine**. Remember to place the barstool on the side of your pullup bar so that the tension from the rope engages the leverage design of the pullup bar. Sit on the barstool with your legs straddling the pulley and PVC handle rope. Grasp the PVC handle with your palm facing up. Keep your back straight and elbow slightly bent.

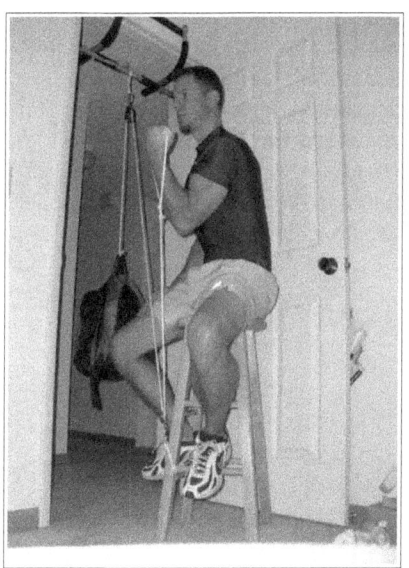

21b. With your back straight slowly raise the handle engaging your bicep muscle. Stop when your forearm is just short of perpendicular to the floor. Pause briefly and slowly return to the starting position. That is 1 rep.

Cross Over Twist (assisted)

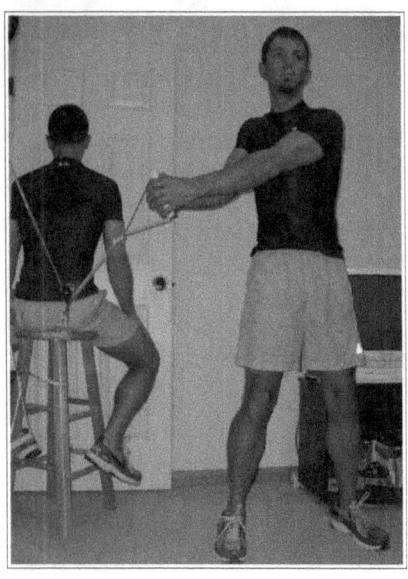

22a. Assemble the **Seated Curling/Lateral Raise Machine** and raise the pulley to the top of the barstool leg just beneath the seat. Remember to place the barstool on the side of your pullup bar so that the tension from the rope engages the leverage design of the pullup bar. Have someone sit on the barstool to keep it from tipping. Grasp the PVC handle with both hands. Keep your back straight and elbows slightly bent and feet shoulder width apart.

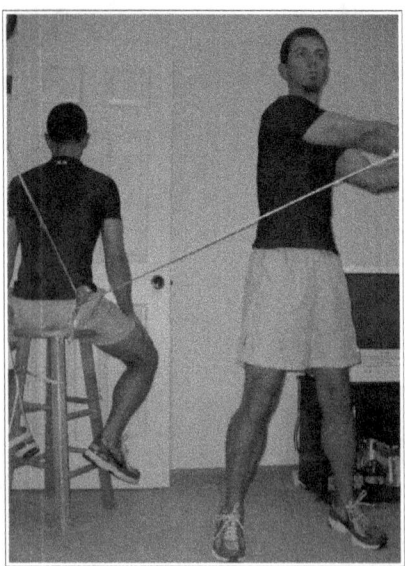

22b. Keeping your elbows slightly bent swiftly pull the PVC handle across your upper torso engaging your abdominal muscles and pectoral muscles. Pause briefly and slowly return to the starting position and feel the stretch in your chest. That is 1 rep.

Cross Over Twist (solo)

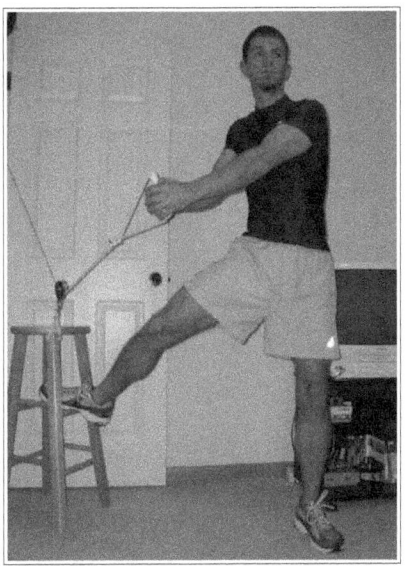

23a. Assemble the **Seated Curling/Lateral Raise Machine** and raise the pulley to the top of the barstool leg just beneath the seat. Remember to place the barstool on the side of your pullup bar so that the tension from the rope engages the leverage design of the pullup bar. Place your foot on the top rung of your barstool supports being careful to maintain your balance. Grasp the PVC handle with both hands. Keep your back straight and elbows slightly bent.

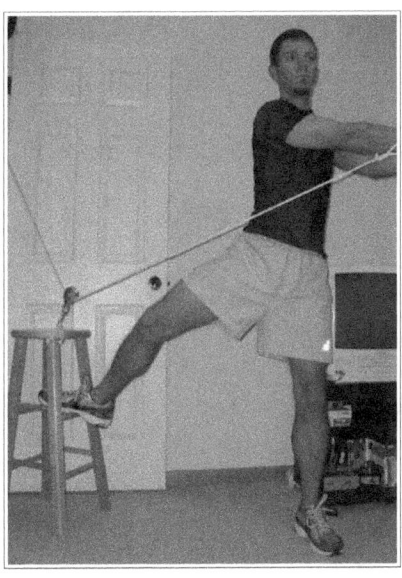

23b. Keeping your elbows slightly bent swiftly pull the pvc handle across your upper torso engaging your abdominal muscles and pectoral muscles. Pause briefly and slowly return to the starting position and feel the stretch in your chest. That is 1 rep.

Dumbbell Bicep Curls

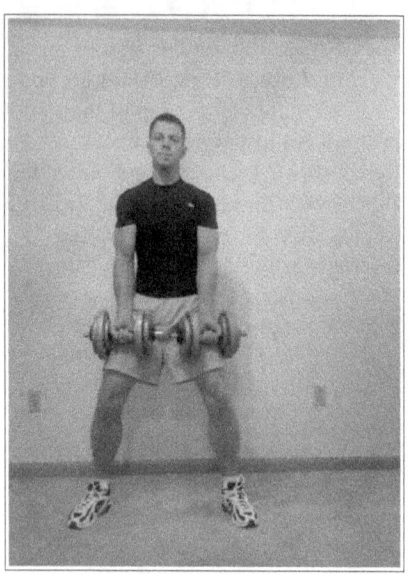

24a. Grasp two dumbbells with your palms facing away from your body. Stand upright keeping your back straight, feet slightly wider than shoulder width apart, and knees slightly bent.

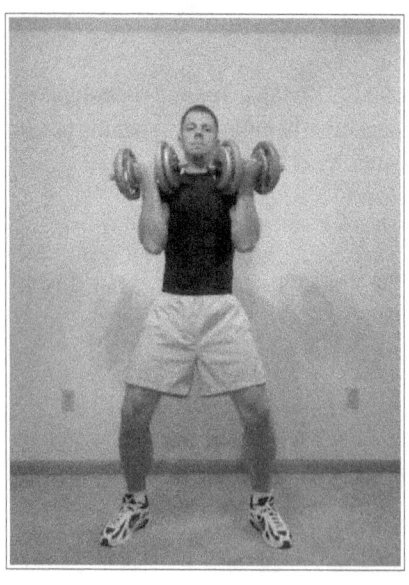

24b. With your back straight and knees slightly bent slowly raise the dumbbells engaging your bicep muscles. Stop when your forearms are just short of perpendicular to the floor or the dumbbells are touching your chest or shoulders. Pause briefly and slowly return to starting position. That is 1 rep.

Note: Don't swing the dumbbells up and don't allow them to fall too quickly when returning to the starting position.

Exercise Ball Dumbbell Press

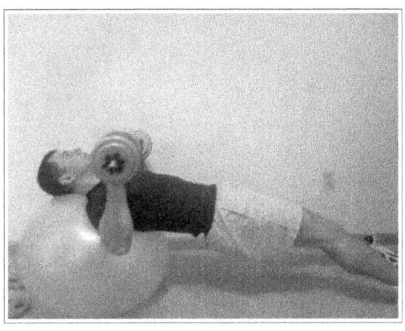 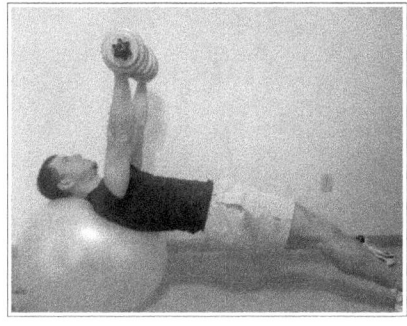

25a. Grasp two dumbbells with your palms facing down and sit on top of your exercise ball. Raise the dumbbells to shoulder height while remaining seated on top of the exercise ball. Slowly roll the exercise ball forward as you walk your feet away from the ball keeping them at least shoulder width apart. Stop when the curve of the ball is positioned under the back of your head, neck, and upper back. Your legs and body should be as straight as possible.

25b. With your body straight ensure that the ball doesn't roll. Slowly push the dumbbells up and away from your body until your arms are just short of straight. Pause briefly and slowly lower the dumbbells to the starting position. That is 1 rep.

Chapter 8

"Chop Some Wood"

Break some bored-s

Now that the flame has been kindled and we've gathered the logs which are necessary for a successful long burning fire, let's chop those logs into manageable pieces and get the fire roaring!

In the previous chapter I laid out over 20 different exercise moves which utilize the full potential of the Backpack Gym and embrace the concept of the Invisible Home Gym. However, all of the moves are not necessary for the basic workout routine I set out to develop when I began my quest to develop the Backpack Gym. In fact each daily workout will only incorporate a few of the moves.

The purpose of providing you with a library of so many exercise moves is to give you the tools not only necessary to build lean muscle mass, but to also help deal with a couple of the major issues that I deal with when it comes to sticking to an exercise program: boredom and the results plateau.

After we get beyond the initial reservations, uncertainties, and fears and we decide to take the leap and begin a new exercise program the initial weeks of the program can be rather exciting.

Our muscles hurt in a good way. We feel energized and fresh. The psychological effects of eating healthy encourage us to push harder and go farther. Stress levels are decreased. We can literally feel the fat melting away. However, if we continue the same routine day in and day out all of the excitement and energy will soon fade away as boredom and discouragement creep in when the results that were pouring in at the beginning slow to a drip.

"Break Some Bored-s"

So to beat the boredom and keep the results stream flowing we will keep the daily workouts to as few exercises as possible and mix them up often. And as your fitness level improves you will find a renewed sense of accomplishment as you increase the amount of weight you are working with and the number of minutes you can spend doing the cardio portion of your workout.

For me, when I hit my target weight-loss and muscle mass I set new goals to keep the excitement fresh. For instance I began to run farther and faster and eventually entered a race which increased the motivation factor exponentially.

Additionally, as you increase the amount of time you spend doing cardio you will want to mix in some cardio variety. One such way to accomplish this while avoiding the need to have to run for longer periods of time is to include interval training in your runs.

For instance if you plan on running for 10 minutes run for 5 minutes within your Fitness HR Zone then increase the intensity for 30 seconds to 1 minute and then drop back down into your Fat Burning/Fitness HR Zone for 1 minute then increase the intensity for 30 seconds to 1 minute and then drop back down. Repeat these intervals for the remainder of your run and adjust times according to your personal fitness level.

When exercising to lose weight it is imperative that you include cardiovascular exercise within your regular workouts. And to achieve maximum results it's important to target those problem areas immediately following the cardio portion of your workout.

For instance if your problem area is your stomach and your cardio consists of a 15 minute run, rest no more than 1 or 2 minutes immediately following your run before moving to your abdominal exercise such as the exercise ball weighted situps/crunches.

Speaking of abdominal exercises, since the purpose of this book is to provide you with a home gym solution that will fit into the smallest of living spaces I searched for an abdominal exercise that mimicked an inclined situp bench as closely as possible.

The inclined rotating situp while holding a weight such as a medicine ball over my head provides the best workout for my abs and when I was going to the gym early on I would perform this move following my runs. To perform this move begin by holding the medicine ball and lying back on the inclined bench and extend the ball above your head. Raise the medicine ball as you sit up. Then lean back rotating the ball to the right (arms extended) and return to the situp position. Then lean back rotating the ball to the left and return to the situp position. Finally, return to the starting position. Since this is my favorite gym exercise to work my abs and I don't have the space in my home for an inclined bench, I sought a comparable option for my small space and the weighted exercise ball situp/crunch fit the bill quite nicely.

Below I've put together a sample 6 week workout schedule and included exercises and duration that should be accessible for the beginner. If you find that the number of repetitions or sets are too high, please adjust for your personal needs, although I wouldn't suggest doing less than 2 sets of exercises for those routines I've suggested a 3 set routine. And as your fitness level improves or if you find that the suggested exercises are too easy or become too easy, please replace the "easy" exercise with a more advanced version of the move. For instance as your upper body strength increases you might want to replace the Abdominal Wide Grip Pullup with the Extreme Weighted Wide Grip Pullup for at least one set.

As you work your way through the 6 week program you'll notice that the beginning of the 4th week brings a new combination of exercises for the remaining 3 weeks. Again this is only a recommendation and you can form your own program to fit your needs, but I would recommend changing up your routine at least every 2 to 3 weeks to keep things fresh and to keep your muscles from adapting to the same movements which will potentially slow your progress if not halting it completely.

If you find yourself getting bored try substituting a comparable exercise in place of your regular, boring exercise. For instance try replacing standard leg raises with the plank position or vice versa.

Another quick fix for boredom is to add an extra rest day between workouts so that you have 2 rest days between exercise days.

Something that I overlooked when I first began my quest to lose weight and improve my health is the importance of rest. I can't stress it enough. Be sure you are getting plenty of sleep at night. If at all possible get a full 8 hours of sleep or more, especially on nights following more strenuous exercise. And to avoid injury be sure to get enough rest days in between exercise day. It can be easy to chase the carrot and think you are helping yourself by exercising 24 hours a day 7 days a week, but in reality you are doing yourself more harm than good.

With that, let's chop some wood!

To begin I've laid out a simple routine that I use as the core of my workout and it is in fact the inspiration behind the Barstool Body Backpack Gym and Invisible Home Gym.

Sharpen the Ax

	Weekly
Day1	15 minutes of cardio performing in your Fitness HR Zone. Mix in intervals of 30 seconds to 1 minute of increased intensity at least once a week. *Exercise ball or weighted exercise ball situps, 1 set of 35 to 50 reps. Standard leg raises using the leg raise/dip machine or Bicep leg raises using the pullup bar. 3 sets of 15 to 20 reps.
Day2	Wide grip pullups or abdominal wide grip pullups. 3 sets as follows. 1 set of 20 reps, 1 set of 10 to 15 reps, 1 set of 10 to 15 reps. Abdominal or standard dips, 3 sets of 10 to 15 reps. Diamond pushups or elevated diamond pushups. 3 sets. 1 set is defined as the number reps you can do without breaking form, or until you begin to arch your back, or you begin to bend your knees.

Day3	**Rest Day or Cardio Only (increase to 20 to 30 minutes)
Day4	Rest Day or Cardio Only (increase to 20 to 30 minutes)
	Repeat

*Rest 1 minute between exercises and 30 seconds to 1 minute between sets.
**You must rest at least one full day. You may choose to rest two days between your longer cardio day and the next regular exercise day.

The above schedule is simply a recommendation for a template that has been very effective for me. In addition to this standard template you will want to include at least 3 days of cardiovascular training per week where you perform within your Fitness HR Zone. Finally, to add a little more wood to the fire on your non-abdominal focused days, you might throw in a set or two of Plank Position isometric exercises while you are watching TV!

Sample Beginner's Workout

	Week 1	Week 2
Day 1	5 to 10 minutes of cardio performing in your Fitness HR Zone. *1 set of 35 ergonomic situps/crunches or ergonomic twist situps/crunches. 3 sets of standard leg raises 15 to 20 reps.	5 to 10 minutes of cardio performing in your Fitness HR Zone. 3 sets of 10 reps standard pullups or pullup training. 3 sets of diamond pushups 3 sets of 8 to 10 reps bicep curls.
Day 2	5 to 10 minutes of cardio performing in your Fitness HR Zone. 3 sets of 10 reps standard pullups or pullup training. 3 sets of diamond pushups 3 sets of 8 to 10 reps bicep curls.	Rest Day

Day3	Rest Day	5 to 10 minutes of cardio performing in your Fitness HR Zone. 1 set of 35 ergonomic situps/crunches or ergonomic twist situps/crunches. 3 sets of standard leg raises 15 to 20 reps.
Day4	5 to 10 minutes of cardio performing in your Fitness HR Zone. 1 set of 35 ergonomic situps/crunches or ergonomic twist situps/crunches. 3 sets of standard leg raises 15 to 20 reps.	5 to 10 minutes of cardio performing in your Fitness HR Zone. 3 sets of 10 reps standard pullups or pullup training. 3 sets of diamond pushups 3 sets of 8 to 10 reps bicep curls.
Day5	5 to 10 minutes of cardio performing in your Fitness HR Zone. 3 sets of 10 reps standard pullups or pullup training. 3 sets of diamond pushups. 3 sets of 8 to 10 reps bicep curls.	Rest Day
Day6	Rest Day	5 to 10 minutes of cardio performing in your Fitness HR Zone. 1 set of 35 ergonomic situps/crunches or ergonomic twist situps/crunches. 3 sets of standard leg raises 15 to 20 reps.
Day7	5 to 10 minutes of cardio performing in your Fitness HR Zone. 1 set of 35 ergonomic situps/crunches or ergonomic twist situps/crunches. 3 sets of standard leg raises 15 to 20 reps.	5 to 10 minutes of cardio performing in your Fitness HR Zone. 3 sets of 10 reps standard pullups or pullup training. 3 sets of diamond pushups 3 sets of 8 to 10 reps bicep curls.

*Rest 1 minute between exercises and 30 seconds to 1 minute between sets.

	Week 3	Week 4
Day1	Rest Day	10 to 15 minutes of cardio performing in your Fitness HR Zone. 3 sets of 10 to 15 reps, Abdominal dips. 3 sets of 10 to 15 reps, pullup training OR abdominal pullups. 3 sets of 15 reps, standard leg raises.
Day2	5 to 10 minutes of cardio performing in your Fitness HR Zone. 1 set of 35 ergonomic situps/crunches or ergonomic twist situps/crunches. 3 sets of standard leg raises 15 to 20 reps.	10 to 15 minutes of cardio performing in your Fitness HR Zone. 3 sets of elevated pushups or elevated diamond pushups. 3 sets of 10 to 15 reps, cable crossover chest flex. 3 sets of 10 to 15 reps, seated lateral raises
Day3	5 to 10 minutes of cardio performing in your Fitness HR Zone. 3 sets of 10 reps standard pullups or pullup training. 3 sets of diamond pushups 3 sets of 8 to 10 reps bicep curls each arm.	Rest Day
Day4	Rest Day	10 to 15 minutes of cardio performing in your Fitness HR Zone. 3 sets of 10 to 15 reps, Abdominal dips. 3 sets of 10 to 15 reps, pullup training OR abdominal pullups. 3 sets of 15 reps, standard leg raises.

Day5	5 to 10 minutes of cardio performing in your Fitness HR Zone. 1 set of 35 ergonomic situps/crunches or ergonomic twist situps/crunches. 3 sets of standard leg raises 15 to 20 reps.	10 to 15 minutes of cardio performing in your Fitness HR Zone. 3 sets of elevated pushups or elevated diamond pushups. 3 sets of 10 to 15 reps, cable crossover chest flex. 3 sets of 10 to 15 reps, seated lateral raises
Day6	5 to 10 minutes of cardio performing in your Fitness HR Zone. 3 sets of 10 reps standard pullups or pullup training. 3 sets of diamond pushups 3 sets of 8 to 10 reps bicep curls each arm.	Rest Day
Day7	Rest Day	10 to 15 minutes of cardio performing in your Fitness HR Zone. 3 sets of 10 to 15 reps, Abdominal dips. 3 sets of 10 to 15 reps, pullup training OR abdominal pullups. 3 sets of 15 reps, standard leg raises.

	Week 5	Week 6
Day1	10 to 15 minutes of cardio performing in your Fitness HR Zone. 3 sets of elevated pushups or elevated diamond pushups. 3 sets of 10 to 15 reps, cable crossover chest flex. 3 sets of 10 to 15 reps, seated lateral raises	Rest Day

Day2	Rest Day	10 to 15 minutes of cardio performing in your Fitness HR Zone. 3 sets of 10 to 15 reps, Abdominal dips. 3 sets of 10 to 15 reps, pullup training OR abdominal pullups. 3 sets of 15 reps, standard leg raises.
Day3	10 to 15 minutes of cardio performing in your Fitness HR Zone. 3 sets of 10 to 15 reps, Abdominal dips. 3 sets of 10 to 15 reps, pullup training OR abdominal pullups. 3 sets of 15 reps, standard leg raises.	10 to 15 minutes of cardio performing in your Fitness HR Zone. 3 sets of elevated pushups or elevated diamond pushups. 3 sets of 10 to 15 reps, cable crossover chest flex. 3 sets of 10 to 15 reps, seated lateral raises
Day4	10 to 15 minutes of cardio performing in your Fitness HR Zone. 3 sets of elevated pushups or elevated diamond pushups. 3 sets of 10 to 15 reps, cable crossover chest flex. 3 sets of 10 to 15 reps, seated lateral raises	Rest Day
Day5	Rest Day	10 to 15 minutes of cardio performing in your Fitness HR Zone. 3 sets of 10 to 15 reps, Abdominal dips. 3 sets of 10 to 15 reps, pullup training OR abdominal pullups. 3 sets of 15 reps, standard leg raises.

Day 6	10 to 15 minutes of cardio performing in your Fitness HR Zone.	10 to 15 minutes of cardio performing in your Fitness HR Zone.
	3 sets of 10 to 15 reps, Abdominal dips.	3 sets of elevated pushups or elevated diamond pushups.
	3 sets of 10 to 15 reps, pullup training OR abdominal pullups.	3 sets of 10 to 15 reps, cable crossover chest flex.
	3 sets of 15 reps, standard leg raises.	3 sets of 10 to 15 reps, seated lateral raises
Day 7	10 to 15 minutes of cardio performing in your Fitness HR Zone.	Rest Day
	3 sets of elevated pushups or elevated diamond pushups.	
	3 sets of 10 to 15 reps, cable crossover chest flex.	
	3 sets of 10 to 15 reps, seated lateral raises	

In closing I want to congratulate you on your choice to make a change in your lifestyle habits and for realizing that things don't have to stay the way they are forever. It is my hope and my desire that the preceding pages have helped to solidify that realization and that your eyes have been opened to at least one new concept that will help you along the journey to a healthier happier you!

I realize the journey is not going to be an easy one, but as I mentioned earlier it is that first step that is always the most difficult. And now that you've begun it will only get easier from here. That's not to say it will ever be easy, if it does you're not pushing yourself to your full potential, but it does become a part of your routine and eventually a part of who you are. You will be making healthy lifestyle choices without even thinking about it and occasionally you'll catch a glimpse of that person you used to be and won't even recognize it was you.

"One final thought. "

As you build lean muscle mass and as your strength and endurance increase you will want to modify the workouts to fit your new fitness levels. This will include adding more weight to your strength training exercises such as wearing the sandbag filled backpack and increasing the amount of time you spend on your cardio sessions. However, it shouldn't be necessary to spend more than 15 or 20 minutes on cardio...we are wanting to keep our daily investment in exercise to a minimum. And remember you can maximize your cardio by substituting interval training in place of your normally paced workouts. Additionally, you will want to reassess your target heart rate zones and modify your cardio workouts accordingly.

Appendix

Resources Consulted

Men's Health. Total Fitness Guide 2007. Printed in the United States of America: Rodale Inc., 2007.

Daniela Hernandez: Los Angeles Times. Study Links Potatoes To Weight Gain. Knoxville News Sentinel. Sunday; June 26, 2011.

Hogen, Dieter: Health Radar. Vol. 1, Issue 6. The Damage a Doughnut Does. A Publication of NewsmaxHealth.com, June 2011.

http://www.usatriathlon.org/about-multisport/multisport-zone/multisport-lab/articles/five-ways-to-blast-your-competition.aspx

http://www.bicycling.com/training-nutrition/nutrition-weight-loss/big-fat-lies

http://fitbie.msn.com/lose-weight/how-pack-15-pounds-muscle

http://fitbie.msn.com/lose-weight/tips/golden-rules-weight-loss/tip/3

http://www.active.com/fitness/Articles/Calculate_your_training_heart_rate_zones.htm

http://www.active.com/women/Articles/How_to_Use_a_Heart_Rate_Monitor.htm

http://www.active.com/nutrition/Articles/Sports-Nutrition-Tips-to-Help-You-Lose-Weight-and-Perform-Better.htm

http://running.about.com/od/howtorun/ht/Calculate-Your-Target-Heart-Rate-Zone.htm

http://en.wikipedia.org/wiki/Heart_rate

http://completerunning.com/archives/2006/10/27/the-karvonen-method-heart-rate-zones/

http://completerunning.com/archives/2006/10/24/slow-down-you-movetoo-fast/

http://forum.bodybuilding.com/showthread.php?t=211647&page=1

http://www.exrx.net/WeightExercises/PectoralSternal/AsChestDip.html

http://stronglifts.com/how-to-perform-dips-with-proper-technique/

Target Heart Rate Zones

The following table is provided to help you determine your optimal target heart rate zones according to the Alternative Method formulas described in Chapter 4. The formulas are based off of an Age Predicted Maximum Heart Rate which is determined by subtracting your age from the number 220. Therefore the "Age" column has been provided as a reference for you to quickly locate your target heart rate zones. If, however, your physician helped you determine your Maximum Heart Rate by performing a cardio stress test or other evaluation, the table will still provide you with a reference to quickly find your target heart rate zones. Simply ignore the "Age" column and locate your maximum heart rate value in the "Age Predicted Max HR" column. Then locate the row containing your "Resting Heart Rate" and the zones listed in that row will be your target heart rate zones, regardless of what "Age" is listed in that same row.

Age	Age Predicted Max HR	Resting Heart Rate	Heart Rate Reserve	Fat Burning Zone Low	Fat Burning High/Fitness Zone Low	Fitness Zone High
18	202	60	142	131	167	181
18	202	65	137	134	168	181
18	202	70	132	136	169	182
18	202	75	127	139	170	183
18	202	80	122	141	172	184
18	202	85	117	144	173	184
18	202	90	112	146	174	185
18	202	95	107	149	175	186
18	202	100	102	151	177	187
19	201	60	141	131	166	180

Age	Age Predicted Max HR	Resting Heart Rate	Heart Rate Reserve	Fat Burning Zone Low	Fat Burning High/Fitness Zone Low	Fitness Zone High
19	201	65	136	133	167	181
19	201	70	131	136	168	181
19	201	75	126	138	170	182
19	201	80	121	141	171	183
19	201	85	116	143	172	184
19	201	90	111	146	173	184
19	201	95	106	148	175	185
19	201	100	101	151	176	186
20	200	60	140	130	165	179
20	200	65	135	133	166	180
20	200	70	130	135	168	181
20	200	75	125	138	169	181
20	200	80	120	140	170	182
20	200	85	115	143	171	183
20	200	90	110	145	173	184
20	200	95	105	148	174	184
20	200	100	100	150	175	185
21	199	60	139	130	164	178
21	199	65	134	132	166	179
21	199	70	129	135	167	180
21	199	75	124	137	168	180
21	199	80	119	140	169	181
21	199	85	114	142	171	182
21	199	90	109	145	172	183
21	199	95	104	147	173	183
21	199	100	99	150	174	184
22	198	60	138	129	164	177
22	198	65	133	132	165	178
22	198	70	128	134	166	179
22	198	75	123	137	167	180
22	198	80	118	139	169	180
22	198	85	113	142	170	181
22	198	90	108	144	171	182
22	198	95	103	147	172	183
22	198	100	98	149	174	183
23	197	60	137	129	163	176
23	197	65	132	131	164	177
23	197	70	127	134	165	178
23	197	75	122	136	167	179
23	197	80	117	139	168	179
23	197	85	112	141	169	180
23	197	90	107	144	170	181
23	197	95	102	146	172	182
23	197	100	97	149	173	182
24	196	60	136	128	162	176
24	196	65	131	131	163	176
24	196	70	126	133	165	177

Age	Age Predicted Max HR	Resting Heart Rate	Heart Rate Reserve	Fat Burning Zone Low	Fat Burning High/Fitness Zone Low	Fitness Zone High
24	196	75	121	136	166	178
24	196	80	116	138	167	179
24	196	85	111	141	168	179
24	196	90	106	143	170	180
24	196	95	101	146	171	181
24	196	100	96	148	172	182
25	195	60	135	128	161	175
25	195	65	130	130	163	176
25	195	70	125	133	164	176
25	195	75	120	135	165	177
25	195	80	115	138	166	178
25	195	85	110	140	168	179
25	195	90	105	143	169	179
25	195	95	100	145	170	180
25	195	100	95	148	171	181
26	194	60	134	127	161	174
26	194	65	129	130	162	175
26	194	70	124	132	163	175
26	194	75	119	135	164	176
26	194	80	114	137	166	177
26	194	85	109	140	167	178
26	194	90	104	142	168	178
26	194	95	99	145	169	179
26	194	100	94	147	171	180
27	193	60	133	127	160	173
27	193	65	128	129	161	174
27	193	70	123	132	162	175
27	193	75	118	134	164	175
27	193	80	113	137	165	176
27	193	85	108	139	166	177
27	193	90	103	142	167	178
27	193	95	98	144	169	178
27	193	100	93	147	170	179
28	192	60	132	126	159	172
28	192	65	127	129	160	173
28	192	70	122	131	162	174
28	192	75	117	134	163	174
28	192	80	112	136	164	175
28	192	85	107	139	165	176
28	192	90	102	141	167	177
28	192	95	97	144	168	177
28	192	100	92	146	169	178
29	191	60	131	126	158	171
29	191	65	126	128	160	172
29	191	70	121	131	161	173
29	191	75	116	133	162	174
29	191	80	111	136	163	174

Age	Age Predicted Max HR	Resting Heart Rate	Heart Rate Reserve	Fat Burning Zone Low	Fat Burning High/Fitness Zone Low	Fitness Zone High
29	191	85	106	138	165	175
29	191	90	101	141	166	176
29	191	95	96	143	167	177
29	191	100	91	146	168	177
30	190	60	130	125	158	171
30	190	65	125	128	159	171
30	190	70	120	130	160	172
30	190	75	115	133	161	173
30	190	80	110	135	163	174
30	190	85	105	138	164	174
30	190	90	100	140	165	175
30	190	95	95	143	166	176
30	190	100	90	145	168	177
31	189	60	129	125	157	170
31	189	65	124	127	158	170
31	189	70	119	130	159	171
31	189	75	114	132	161	172
31	189	80	109	135	162	173
31	189	85	104	137	163	173
31	189	90	99	140	164	174
31	189	95	94	142	166	175
31	189	100	89	145	167	176
32	188	60	128	124	156	169
32	188	65	123	127	157	170
32	188	70	118	129	159	170
32	188	75	113	132	160	171
32	188	80	108	134	161	172
32	188	85	103	137	162	173
32	188	90	98	139	164	173
32	188	95	93	142	165	174
32	188	100	88	144	166	175
33	187	60	127	124	155	168
33	187	65	122	126	157	169
33	187	70	117	129	158	169
33	187	75	112	131	159	170
33	187	80	107	134	160	171
33	187	85	102	136	162	172
33	187	90	97	139	163	172
33	187	95	92	141	164	173
33	187	100	87	144	165	174
34	186	60	126	123	155	167
34	186	65	121	126	156	168
34	186	70	116	128	157	169
34	186	75	111	131	158	169
34	186	80	106	133	160	170
34	186	85	101	136	161	171
34	186	90	96	138	162	172

Age	Age Predicted Max HR	Resting Heart Rate	Heart Rate Reserve	Fat Burning Zone Low	Fat Burning High/Fitness Zone Low	Fitness Zone High
34	186	95	91	141	163	172
34	186	100	86	143	165	173
35	185	60	125	123	154	166
35	185	65	120	125	155	167
35	185	70	115	128	156	168
35	185	75	110	130	158	169
35	185	80	105	133	159	169
35	185	85	100	135	160	170
35	185	90	95	138	161	171
35	185	95	90	140	163	172
35	185	100	85	143	164	172
36	184	60	124	122	153	165
36	184	65	119	125	154	166
36	184	70	114	127	156	167
36	184	75	109	130	157	168
36	184	80	104	132	158	168
36	184	85	99	135	159	169
36	184	90	94	137	161	170
36	184	95	89	140	162	171
36	184	100	84	142	163	171
37	183	60	123	122	152	165
37	183	65	118	124	154	165
37	183	70	113	127	155	166
37	183	75	108	129	156	167
37	183	80	103	132	157	168
37	183	85	98	134	159	168
37	183	90	93	137	160	169
37	183	95	88	139	161	170
37	183	100	83	142	162	171
38	182	60	122	121	152	164
38	182	65	117	124	153	164
38	182	70	112	126	154	165
38	182	75	107	129	155	166
38	182	80	102	131	157	167
38	182	85	97	134	158	167
38	182	90	92	136	159	168
38	182	95	87	139	160	169
38	182	100	82	141	162	170
39	181	60	121	121	151	163
39	181	65	116	123	152	164
39	181	70	111	126	153	164
39	181	75	106	128	155	165
39	181	80	101	131	156	166
39	181	85	96	133	157	167
39	181	90	91	136	158	167
39	181	95	86	138	160	168
39	181	100	81	141	161	169

Age	Age Predicted Max HR	Resting Heart Rate	Heart Rate Reserve	Fat Burning Zone Low	Fat Burning High/Fitness Zone Low	Fitness Zone High
40	180	60	120	120	150	162
40	180	65	115	123	151	163
40	180	70	110	125	153	164
40	180	75	105	128	154	164
40	180	80	100	130	155	165
40	180	85	95	133	156	166
40	180	90	90	135	158	167
40	180	95	85	138	159	167
40	180	100	80	140	160	168
41	179	60	119	120	149	161
41	179	65	114	122	151	162
41	179	70	109	125	152	163
41	179	75	104	127	153	163
41	179	80	99	130	154	164
41	179	85	94	132	156	165
41	179	90	89	135	157	166
41	179	95	84	137	158	166
41	179	100	79	140	159	167
42	178	60	118	119	149	160
42	178	65	113	122	150	161
42	178	70	108	124	151	162
42	178	75	103	127	152	163
42	178	80	98	129	154	163
42	178	85	93	132	155	164
42	178	90	88	134	156	165
42	178	95	83	137	157	166
42	178	100	78	139	159	166
43	177	60	117	119	148	159
43	177	65	112	121	149	160
43	177	70	107	124	150	161
43	177	75	102	126	152	162
43	177	80	97	129	153	162
43	177	85	92	131	154	163
43	177	90	87	134	155	164
43	177	95	82	136	157	165
43	177	100	77	139	158	165
44	176	60	116	118	147	159
44	176	65	111	121	148	159
44	176	70	106	123	150	160
44	176	75	101	126	151	161
44	176	80	96	128	152	162
44	176	85	91	131	153	162
44	176	90	86	133	155	163
44	176	95	81	136	156	164
44	176	100	76	138	157	165
45	175	60	115	118	146	158
45	175	65	110	120	148	159

Age	Age Predicted Max HR	Resting Heart Rate	Heart Rate Reserve	Fat Burning Zone Low	Fat Burning High/Fitness Zone Low	Fitness Zone High
45	175	70	105	123	149	159
45	175	75	100	125	150	160
45	175	80	95	128	151	161
45	175	85	90	130	153	162
45	175	90	85	133	154	162
45	175	95	80	135	155	163
45	175	100	75	138	156	164
46	174	60	114	117	146	157
46	174	65	109	120	147	158
46	174	70	104	122	148	158
46	174	75	99	125	149	159
46	174	80	94	127	151	160
46	174	85	89	130	152	161
46	174	90	84	132	153	161
46	174	95	79	135	154	162
46	174	100	74	137	156	163
47	173	60	113	117	145	156
47	173	65	108	119	146	157
47	173	70	103	122	147	158
47	173	75	98	124	149	158
47	173	80	93	127	150	159
47	173	85	88	129	151	160
47	173	90	83	132	152	161
47	173	95	78	134	154	161
47	173	100	73	137	155	162
48	172	60	112	116	144	155
48	172	65	107	119	145	156
48	172	70	102	121	147	157
48	172	75	97	124	148	157
48	172	80	92	126	149	158
48	172	85	87	129	150	159
48	172	90	82	131	152	160
48	172	95	77	134	153	160
48	172	100	72	136	154	161
49	171	60	111	116	143	154
49	171	65	106	118	145	155
49	171	70	101	121	146	156
49	171	75	96	123	147	157
49	171	80	91	126	148	157
49	171	85	86	128	150	158
49	171	90	81	131	151	159
49	171	95	76	133	152	160
49	171	100	71	136	153	160
50	170	60	110	115	143	154
50	170	65	105	118	144	154
50	170	70	100	120	145	155
50	170	75	95	123	146	156

Age	Age Predicted Max HR	Resting Heart Rate	Heart Rate Reserve	Fat Burning Zone Low	Fat Burning High/Fitness Zone Low	Fitness Zone High
50	170	80	90	125	148	157
50	170	85	85	128	149	157
50	170	90	80	130	150	158
50	170	95	75	133	151	159
50	170	100	70	135	153	160
51	169	60	109	115	142	153
51	169	65	104	117	143	153
51	169	70	99	120	144	154
51	169	75	94	122	146	155
51	169	80	89	125	147	156
51	169	85	84	127	148	156
51	169	90	79	130	149	157
51	169	95	74	132	151	158
51	169	100	69	135	152	159
52	168	60	108	114	141	152
52	168	65	103	117	142	153
52	168	70	98	119	144	153
52	168	75	93	122	145	154
52	168	80	88	124	146	155
52	168	85	83	127	147	156
52	168	90	78	129	149	156
52	168	95	73	132	150	157
52	168	100	68	134	151	158
53	167	60	107	114	140	151
53	167	65	102	116	142	152
53	167	70	97	119	143	152
53	167	75	92	121	144	153
53	167	80	87	124	145	154
53	167	85	82	126	147	155
53	167	90	77	129	148	155
53	167	95	72	131	149	156
53	167	100	67	134	150	157
54	166	60	106	113	140	150
54	166	65	101	116	141	151
54	166	70	96	118	142	152
54	166	75	91	121	143	152
54	166	80	86	123	145	153
54	166	85	81	126	146	154
54	166	90	76	128	147	155
54	166	95	71	131	148	155
54	166	100	66	133	150	156
55	165	60	105	113	139	149
55	165	65	100	115	140	150
55	165	70	95	118	141	151
55	165	75	90	120	143	152
55	165	80	85	123	144	152
55	165	85	80	125	145	153

95

Age	Age Predicted Max HR	Resting Heart Rate	Heart Rate Reserve	Fat Burning Zone Low	Fat Burning High/Fitness Zone Low	Fitness Zone High
55	165	90	75	128	146	154
55	165	95	70	130	148	155
55	165	100	65	133	149	155
56	164	60	104	112	138	148
56	164	65	99	115	139	149
56	164	70	94	117	141	150
56	164	75	89	120	142	151
56	164	80	84	122	143	151
56	164	85	79	125	144	152
56	164	90	74	127	146	153
56	164	95	69	130	147	154
56	164	100	64	132	148	154
57	163	60	103	112	137	148
57	163	65	98	114	139	148
57	163	70	93	117	140	149
57	163	75	88	119	141	150
57	163	80	83	122	142	151
57	163	85	78	124	144	151
57	163	90	73	127	145	152
57	163	95	68	129	146	153
57	163	100	63	132	147	154
58	162	60	102	111	137	147
58	162	65	97	114	138	147
58	162	70	92	116	139	148
58	162	75	87	119	140	149
58	162	80	82	121	142	150
58	162	85	77	124	143	150
58	162	90	72	126	144	151
58	162	95	67	129	145	152
58	162	100	62	131	147	153
59	161	60	101	111	136	146
59	161	65	96	113	137	147
59	161	70	91	116	138	147
59	161	75	86	118	140	148
59	161	80	81	121	141	149
59	161	85	76	123	142	150
59	161	90	71	126	143	150
59	161	95	66	128	145	151
59	161	100	61	131	146	152
60	160	60	100	110	135	145
60	160	65	95	113	136	146
60	160	70	90	115	138	147
60	160	75	85	118	139	147
60	160	80	80	120	140	148
60	160	85	75	123	141	149
60	160	90	70	125	143	150
60	160	95	65	128	144	150

Age	Age Predicted Max HR	Resting Heart Rate	Heart Rate Reserve	Fat Burning Zone Low	Fat Burning High/Fitness Zone Low	Fitness Zone High
60	160	100	60	130	145	151
61	159	60	99	110	134	144
61	159	65	94	112	136	145
61	159	70	89	115	137	146
61	159	75	84	117	138	146
61	159	80	79	120	139	147
61	159	85	74	122	141	148
61	159	90	69	125	142	149
61	159	95	64	127	143	149
61	159	100	59	130	144	150
62	158	60	98	109	134	143
62	158	65	93	112	135	144
62	158	70	88	114	136	145
62	158	75	83	117	137	146
62	158	80	78	119	139	146
62	158	85	73	122	140	147
62	158	90	68	124	141	148
62	158	95	63	127	142	149
62	158	100	58	129	144	149
63	157	60	97	109	133	142
63	157	65	92	111	134	143
63	157	70	87	114	135	144
63	157	75	82	116	137	145
63	157	80	77	119	138	145
63	157	85	72	121	139	146
63	157	90	67	124	140	147
63	157	95	62	126	142	148
63	157	100	57	129	143	148
64	156	60	96	108	132	142
64	156	65	91	111	133	142
64	156	70	86	113	135	143
64	156	75	81	116	136	144
64	156	80	76	118	137	145
64	156	85	71	121	138	145
64	156	90	66	123	140	146
64	156	95	61	126	141	147
64	156	100	56	128	142	148
65	155	60	95	108	131	141
65	155	65	90	110	133	142
65	155	70	85	113	134	142
65	155	75	80	115	135	143
65	155	80	75	118	136	144
65	155	85	70	120	138	145
65	155	90	65	123	139	145
65	155	95	60	125	140	146
65	155	100	55	128	141	147